3599

WD 460

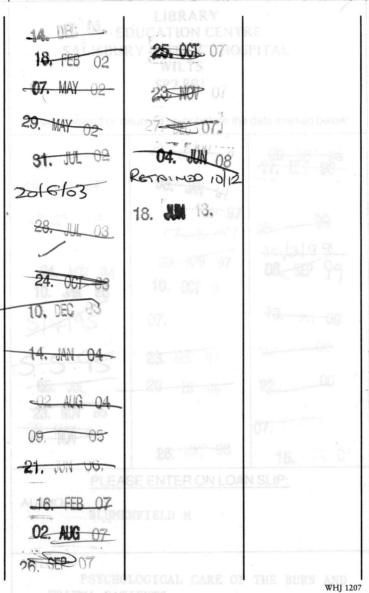

14. DEC 00

18. FEB 02

07. MAY 02

29. MAY 02

31. JUL 02

20/6/03

28. JUL 03

24. OCT 03

10. DEC 03

14. JAN 04

02. AUG 04

09. NOV 05

21. JUN 06

16. FEB 07

02. AUG 07

26. SEP 07

25. OCT 07

23. NOV 07

27. DEC 07

04. JUN 08

RETAINED 10/12

18. JUN 13

WHJ 1207

Books should be returned to the SDH Library on or before
the date stamped above unless a renewal has been arranged.

Salisbury District Hospital Library

Telephone: Salisbury (01722) 336262   extn. 4432 / 33
Out of hours answer machine in operation

Psychological Care
of the Burn and
Trauma Patient

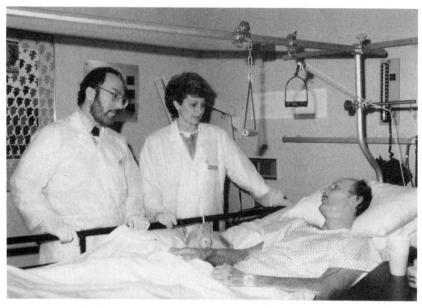

Dr. Blumenfield and Ms. Schoeps speak with a patient.

Psychological Care of the Burn and Trauma Patient

....

MICHAEL BLUMENFIELD, M.D.

Professor of Psychiatry, Medicine and Surgery
Department of Psychiatry and Behavioral Sciences
New York Medical College
Valhalla, New York

MARGOT M. SCHOEPS, M.S., R.N., C.S.

Psychiatric Clinical Nurse-Specialist
Instructor of Psychiatry
New York Medical College
Valhalla, New York

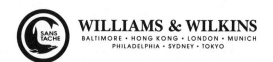

WILLIAMS & WILKINS
BALTIMORE · HONG KONG · LONDON · MUNICH
PHILADELPHIA · SYDNEY · TOKYO

Editor: Michael G. Fisher
Associate Editor: Carol Eckhart
Copy Editor: Dominique van de Stadt
Designer: Norman W. Och
Illustration Planner: Lorraine Wrzosek
Production Coordinator: Barbara J. Felton
Cover Illustration: Gregory J. Vinck

Copyright © 1993
Williams & Wilkins
428 East Preston Street
Baltimore, Maryland 21202, USA

Accurate indications, adverse reactions, and dosage schedules for drugs are provided in this book, but it is possible that they may change. The reader is urged to review the package information data of the manufacturers of the medications mentioned.

Printed in the United States of America

Chapter reprints are available from the Publisher.

Library of Congress Cataloging-in-Publication Data

Blumenfield, Michael.
    Psychological care of the burn and trauma patient / Michael Blumenfield, Margot M. Schoeps.
        p.   cm.
    Includes index.
    ISBN 0-683-00876-5
    1. Wounds and injuries—Psychological aspects. 2. Burns and scalds—Psychological aspects. 3. Wounds and injuries—Patients—Rehabilitation. 4. Burns and scalds—Patients—Rehabilitation. I. Schoeps, Margot M. II. Title.
    [DNLM: 1. Burns—psychology. 2. Psychotherapy—methods. 3. Wounds and Injuries—psychology. WO 704 B658p]
    RD93.B58   1992
    617.1′0019—dc20
    M/DLC
    for Library of Congress   92–5497
                                                                                        CIP

92   93   94   95   96
1   2   3   4   5   6   7   8   9   10

Dedication

To Susan and Fred
and our children
Jay, Bob, Sharon,
Heidi, Mark, Amy

FOREWORD

Only while looking into the well-draped sterile field of the operating room will the burn surgeon forget for a short time the complex psychological factors that affect the patient. At the bedside or in my consulting room, I am intimately aware of the pain, confusion, anxiety, depression, and vast array of human feelings that are brought forth by an unexpected injury.

Each person possesses a unique personality that sometimes includes serious psychological problems. As we care for a burn and trauma patient, the personal side of that man, woman, or child becomes known to us. We learn to appreciate the strengths and weaknesses of families and other relationships that support the patient. It is not our task to understand all of these people, but it is our responsibility to work with them and with our patient toward a successful recovery.

The practice of medicine brings with it a commitment to a lifetime of education. We learn from our patients, from our colleagues, and from the writings of a book such as this. Far too often, we tend to think, to interpret, and to act purely on a mechanistic level. I am particularly pleased with the detailed chapter on pain (Chapter 1) and the guidelines for how to treat this brutal enemy. Pain control is a complex issue that involves sophisticated pharmacology and human psychology.

I remember several years ago when a young child was brought into our unit severely injured by an explosion. There was no hope for survival. I will never forget the look on the parents' faces and the depth of pain that I felt for them. My own child was the same age and I could feel every agonizing emotion that the parents were experiencing. It is very important for all of us in this field to understand how our own feelings and emotions can reverberate as we deal with tragedies in our patients. There are times when these emotions have to be addressed with guidance from professionals such as Michael Blumenfield and Margot Schoeps.

This book will be of value to all who work with burn and trauma patients—psychiatrists, social workers, nurses, and surgeons such as myself. I have had the opportunity to interact with the authors for over 10 years at this medical center. We have discussed many of the topics that they cover and I have had the pleasure of seeing my patients benefit from this expertise, which will be presented in this book.

Roger Salisbury, MD
President American Burn Association
Valhalla, 1992

PREFACE

This book is about the psychological understanding and care of hospitalized burn and trauma patients. It is written for mental health professionals who will venture into this field of practice as well as for the nurses, physicians, and other health care professionals who work in the area of burn and trauma and appreciate the need for a psychological perspective in their work.

Our psychological understanding of burn and trauma patients comes from many years of experience working with these patients and their families as well as from our work in general consultation liaison psychiatry and hospice care. We recognize that every hospital setting is different. There are many issues that we describe that may be unique to a burn patient and that may not always apply to a non-burn, trauma situation. However, much of what we have learned from our work on a burn unit can readily be applied to trauma patients wherever they may be hospitalized.

The common ground for most patients described in this book is that they have experienced a significant trauma that has required their hospitalization and inevitably confronted them with physical pain, anxiety, depression, and uncertainty about the future. Their injuries also brought them into a relationship with the readers of this book—professionals dedicated to the care of burn and trauma patients.

We begin the book with a chapter on pain because pain is the primary issue that must be addressed before other psychological concerns can be considered. We conclude the book with a chapter on psychological support and care of the staff because, although this is a component that is frequently overlooked, it is essential for there to be proper care of the patient.

We wish to recognize our special colleagues with whom we have worked in the burn and trauma setting and who have facilitated our work. This book would not have been possible without Dr. Roger Salisbury and Dr. Jane Petro, the outstanding plastic surgeons who direct the Westchester Burn Center and who have readily welcomed psychological input for their patients. Other very important past and present members of the burn and trauma teams whom we want to acknowledge are doctors Andrew Salzberg,

Sidney Rapp, and John Savino; nurses Mary McMorrow, Tonya Zwirz, Pat Reddish, Connie Conley, and Lauren Johnson; social worker Marie Malone; and occupational therapist Judy Carr-Collins. Equally important are the many nurses, technicians, dietitians, social workers, housestaff, and attending physicians with whom we have worked over the years. Lastly, we want to acknowledge the patients whom we have had the privilege to treat and who are our ultimate teachers.

Michael Blumenfield, M.D.
Margot M. Schoeps, M.S., R.N., C.S.

CONTENTS

1

....

Pain

Several years ago *Life* magazine featured an article about a renowned Burn and Trauma Center where the most technologically advanced care saved many lives. In the article, the head nurse of this medical center, knowing the amount of pain burn patients face, said that if she ever had severe burns she would prefer death over the suffering that goes with the treatment of burns. Unfortunately, we have heard more than one patient at the end of a "successful hospitalization" for severe burn or trauma make similar comments. For this reason, we believe that the issues of pain and pain control must be addressed at the beginning of our book.

Over 75,000,000 traumatic injuries occur every year in the U.S. It is estimated that at least one-third of these result in moderate-to-severe pain (1). It is also estimated that one-third of the more than 5 million critically ill patients managed in intensive care units every year, especially those who are recovering from trauma or surgery, may be expected to suffer episodes of acute pain (2).

Pain control is an issue that must be addressed by every discipline involved in patient care. The physician must assess pain and order the proper medication and dosage as well as its frequency and route of administration. The nurse also makes assessments, delivers medication, and helps to evaluate the effectiveness of the pain management being utilized. Likewise, the physical and occupational therapists have an interest in adequate pain control. The patient cannot carry out prescribed therapy programs unless the pain is controlled. The dietician has another set of problems: Pain medication may cause nausea or so sedate the patient that he or she may be unable to eat to maintain body requirements for healing. Family, friends, and clergy are also part of the care "team," and the support they give is often ineffective if pain is not addressed first.

Pain and pain control are of particular importance to the psychosocial team involved in the patient's care. It is impossible to assess psychological issues such as reaction to injury, depression, guilt, body image, and dementia while the patient has significant pain. A patient in pain has little tolerance for any meaningful conversation. Any effort to talk to the patient without addressing pain status will be experienced by the patient as insensitive and irrelevant. Thus, *during almost every patient contact by a member of our psychosocial team*, we include an inquiry about the adequacy of pain control. One can never assume that this is not a major area of concern for the patient. So often, during the heroic efforts to save the patient's life and retain maximum function of all organ systems, the degree of pain and suffering is neglected by the well-meaning medical and nursing staff.

What Is Pain?

A definition of pain adopted by the International Association for the Study of Pain states that "Pain is an unpleasant sensory and emotional experience associated with an actual or potential tissue damage or described in terms of such damage" (3). Immediate pain may be caused by mechanical or chemical irritation or by tissue damage secondary to trauma, surgery, debridement, physical therapy, ambulation, or any movement. Continuous pain may occur from direct damage or stimulation to the nervous receptors themselves or from stimulation secondary to swelling, edema, tissue movement, and so forth. The anatomical pathways through which pain sensation are carried to the spinothalamic track are fairly well defined and will not be described here. Pain is not merely a sensation to be experienced. Pain carries a complex, real or imagined, subjective component.

In most instances of trauma and burn, the patient not only has an actual physical injury, but is influenced by emotional and subjective variables. There are innumerable factors that account for the amount of pain a patient experiences, and an additional set of variables influences the amount of pain that is expressed. Current theories on pain control postulate that the peripheral sensations of pain can actually be affected by emotions and the psychological state of the person experiencing the pain. The most widely held theory is that of *gate control* (4).

Impulses from pain receptors travel via small and large diameter fibers to the substantia gelatinosa in the dorsal horn of the spinal cord. According to the gate control theory, the impulse can be modulated here by the introduction of medication, the alteration of memories or emotions, or by other influences on the "gate," thus increasing or decreasing the actual transmission of the pain impulses.

Psychological Aspects of Pain

Patients in pain often undergo a psychological regression. They are in a very dependent position and feel great helplessness. Any injury brings up unconscious fears of dying that relate to separation anxiety and intensify the regression. Witnessing other patients in an intensive care unit further exaggerates this fear of dying. Such situations may actually change the pain threshold through the gate mechanism described above. A person may consciously focus on the pain as a symbol of the illness and of the threat to his or her life. The patient may be unconsciously trying to elicit a more caring response from his or her environment. It is for this reason that the doctor-patient/nurse-patient relationship is so important in handling the pain.

This relationship, at a conscious level, can provide comfort as well as tangible relief through medication and procedures. At an unconscious level, the relationship can provide important emotional gratification. A patient who feels isolated and lonely will likely feel anxious and depressed, possibly intensifying the difficulty of controlling his or her pain.

When acute pain, such as postoperative or burn trauma pain, is inadequately managed, the patient can develop a pain symptom complex (5). As this complex evolves, the patient becomes increasingly anxious, depressed, hostile, and lonely, and develops sleep disturbances. Each of these factors exacerbates the perception of pain. Each situation that exacerbates one of these symptoms will subsequently cause increased pain.

It has further been suggested that in a strong social relationship, where the individual has a significant other person such as a marital partner, the treatment of pain can be enhanced with the inclusion of the committed partner in the treatment program (6). This is particularly pertinent to the rehabilitation phase of treatment, when the partner begins to participate in the dressing changes, etc. We have also noted that when family members visit patients in the hospital, the need for pain medication frequently diminishes.

There is an important role for mental health professionals not only in helping the patient deal with his conflicts, conscious and unconscious, but also in overtly teaching the patient strategies for coping with the pain of an acute injury. In one study (7), 20 patients with comparable burn injuries were admitted to a Burn Center and randomly assigned to either a control or an experimental group. The experimental patients received systematic instructions on how to cope with the pain and the stress of the burn injury. The control group only received the standard information that surgical patients are given and social support. Results showed that the experimental group reported less pain and a greater sense of psychological well-being compared to the control group. Moreover, the experimental patients went home, on the average, more than one week sooner than the control patients. The results of this study may have significant implications regarding the economics of medical care—how treatment of pain relates to the DRGs, for example.

The anxiety and depression of a patient in pain may cause psychological responses that complicate the medical condition and thereby intensify the pain. Increased catecholamine release or increased sympathetic neuronal activity also leads to more muscular tension, which will affect pain.

It is important to know the patient's previous experience with pain. People who have had an unpleasant or even traumatic experience with pain in the past will have increased anxiety in the current situation when confronted with pain or the possibility of pain. This anxiety exacerbates the pain experience.

We have found that if the pain is not adequately controlled during the early stages of injury, the patient will develop a psychologically conditioned fear of having pain on movement. Such patients will become immobilized by pain and will be much more difficult to motivate for the exercise activities necessary to achieve a satisfactory range of motion during the rehabilitation phase of an injury. Failure to mobilize the patient when appropriate will then lead to contractures and muscle atrophy. In a similar manner, patients who resist deep breathing or turning because of pain or fear of pain are more prone to infection and pneumonia. They are more likely to have longer hospitalizations, greater morbidity, and perhaps even greater mortality. Their rehabilitations will be more difficult and perhaps less successful.

The psychological approach to the patient in pain must always be supplementary to all efforts to relieve the pain by physical methods such as surgical intervention and pharmacology. The presence of the physician or nurse who is interested in the patient's pain will be very important, as we noted above. It is meaningful to the patient to be reassured that the pain is "legitimate," and that it is temporary and will diminish gradually with recovery (*if* this is in fact true) (8). It is also helpful for the patient to receive information about medication and other interventions that are expected to alleviate the pain as much as possible.

While it is our experience that meaningful psychotherapeutic work cannot be done with an injured patient in acute pain, there are times when one needs to attempt psychological interventions under these conditions because the interventions themselves help to alleviate the pain. For example, patients who blame themselves or other persons may need help to handle these feelings. Learning how to cope with such feelings may alleviate physical pain. These approaches are discussed at a later point in this book.

Measurement of Pain and Communication About Pain

Imagine trying to explain *pain* to a person who never had the sensation. This may be how a burn or trauma patient feels when trying to communicate a degree of pain that most health care workers have never experienced.

There are many methods for measuring and communicating about pain (9–11). Methods of measurement may include subjective reports determined by rating scales or questionnaires, behavioral assessments, or the physiological parameters discussed below. Since most other measurements in health care are objectively determined by scientific criteria, there is an inclination to try to do the same with measurement of pain. But as pain is really a subjective experience, such techniques usually fail. No matter how the various levels of pain are defined, exact, objective criteria for the description of pain are difficult to establish.

We have found that subjective measurement is best to measure pain, and we suggest the Visual Analog Pain Scale (VAPS) (Fig. 1.1) as a suitable method. The Scale shows one line. At the beginning of the line is printed "No pain," and at the end, "Pain as bad as it could be." The caregiver places a mark somewhere along the line, depending on the degree of pain he or she perceives that the patient is experiencing during a procedure. Then the caregiver writes in the kind of medications and pain relief adjuncts that the patient has received and checks off the procedure performed (dressing, debridement, etc.).

A health care worker caring for burn and trauma patients should become familiar with this measurement technique, although it rarely will be used on a daily basis with each patient. VAPS can be monitored and discussed among staff while various interventions are being studied. For example, the patient may be reported to have a VAPS score that diminished from 9.5 to 4.0 during a dressing change, or that rose from 3.0 during the morning to about 5.0 within 2 hours after medication. The absolute value of scores is not very important because it will differ from person to person and only gives an indication of the degree of pain. However, the *changes* in VAPS will show the effectiveness of any interventions and will reflect control or lack of control of the pain. The VAPS score can also be made by the patient

Side 1

Patient form--Visual Analog Pain Scale

#1 Predressing change

No pain [_____/_____] Pain as bad
                                                as it could be

Patient name: *Doe, Jane* Date: *4/23/92* Time: *10:15* a.m.
                                                          p.m.

_____

#2 Postdressing change   (Please fold in half)

No pain [_____/_____] Pain as bad
                                                    as it could be

(Please complete reverse side)

Figure 1.1. Patient form for Visual Analog Pain Scale (Part 1). From Blumenfield M, Reddish P. Burn Unit, Westchester County Medical Center, 1982.

Patient form--Visual Analog Pain Scale   Side 2

Name: _DOE, JANE___ Date: _4/23/82_ Time of dressing _10___ ~~30~~ (a.m.)
                                                          p.m.

Pain and/or psychotropic medications (i.e., Valium,
Thorazine, Vistaril, etc.):

	Medication	Dosage	Route	Time
1.	MORPHINE	10 mg.	I.V.	10^{25}
2.	MORPHINE	10 mg.	I.V.	10^{35}
3.	MORPHINE	10 mg.	I.V.	10^{45}
4.	_____	_____	_____	_____

Other pain, tranquilizer, and/or antidepressant medication:

5. _____   _____   _____   _____

6. _____   _____   _____   _____

Pain relief adjuncts: Procedure (check all that apply:

___ hypnosis   _✓_ burn dressing (i.e., gentle
___ relaxation technique   cleansing and Silvadene)
_✓_ other (specify)_____   ___ adherent dressings, (i.e.,
    DEEP BREATHING   xeroform)
                               ___ wet-dry dressings
                               _✓_ debridement
                               ___ other (specify)_____

Location:

___ patient's room
_✓_ hydrotherapy
___ shower
___ operating room
___ other (specify) _____

Nurse's comments, if any: Pt. ABLE TO ASSIST c̄ CARES TO
    LOWER EXTREMETIES. WOUNDS CLEAN.

Figure 1.1.   Visual Analog Pain Scale (Part 2). From Blumenfield M, Reddish P.
Burn Unit, Westchester County Medical Center, 1982.

at various times under different conditions, and those scores can be compared with the caregivers' scores.

An electronic visual analog apparatus (EVA) (Fig. 1.2) for rapid measurement of a patient's pain has been developed recently. The EVA can be used to communicate about pain when the patient is unable to talk, such as in an intubated state. Even when the patient cannot move his or her hand to mark the line or to move the lever on the EVA, the staff can slowly move along the line until the patient signals a point (Fig. 1.3). This method is reliable and shows consistency when it is repeated under the same circumstances with the same patient.

Even with young children, the drawing of a smiling face at one pole of a line and a sad face at the other pole on the Wong-Baker Faces Pain Scale (Fig. 1.4) allows the child to signal the degree of discomfort.

The specific time periods when these subjective methods of pain measurement are useful are at rest between dressing changes; just prior to the next dressing change; at the start of dressing change, when the dressings

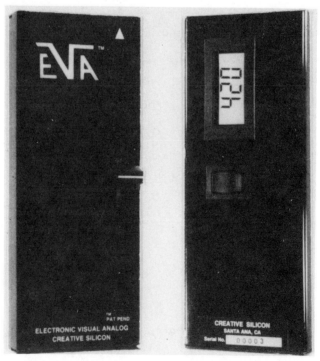

Figure 1.2. Both sides of the Electronic Visual Analog (EVA) Apparatus for measuring pain. Manufactured by Creative Silicon, 2139 North Ross Street, Santa Ana, CA 92706.

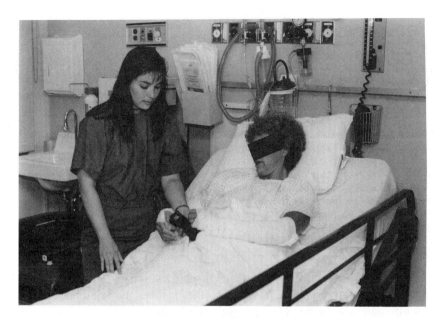

Figure 1.3. Patient utilizing the Visual Analog Pain Scale.

are removed; during the dressing change, when the wounds are debrided; at the end of the dressing change, when the dressing is replaced; during physical therapy or other activities such as ambulation; and during the time allotted for sleep (8).

Patients who have been given long-acting paralyzing agents, particularly during surgery, might have difficulty signaling that they are having pain. In the intensive care unit, the patient may not be able to communicate, often because of intubation. The patient may, however, be agitated, restless, or hyperventilating—all of which are signs of pain. Subtle evidence of pain and anxiety is expressed as tachycardia, hypertension, sweating, and decreased urine output, which occurs due to the increased sympathetic tone. If the patient is intubated and cannot talk, it is essential for him to be able to communicate using a pad and pencil or other methods such as the VAPS or EVA described above. It may be dangerous to rely on the patient's symptoms alone. Hypoxia, for example, may mimic pain and present as agitation, with increased blood pressure and increased heart rate. The administration of a narcotic agent under these conditions could further depress respiration and thus endanger the patient.

Hyperdynamic responses to alcohol and drug withdrawal mimic the presentation of pain. There are situations where the patient could present with

Faces Pain Rating Scale

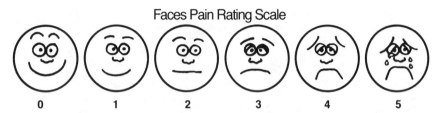

Figure 1.4. Wong-Baker Faces Pain Scale. Explain to the person that each face is for a person who feels happy because he has no pain (hurt) or sad because he has some or a lot of pain. Face 0 is very happy because he doesn't hurt at all. Face 1 hurts just a little bit. Face 2 hurts a little more. Face 3 hurts even more. Face 4 hurts a whole lot. Face 5 hurts as much as you can imagine, although you don't have to be crying to feel this bad. Ask the person to choose the face that best describes how he is feeling. Recommended for persons age 3 years and older. Reproduced by permission from Wong, Donna L., and Whaley, Lucille F. Clinical manual of pediatric nursing, ed. 3, St. Louis, 1990, The C. V. Mosby Co.

both conditions, making determination of pain extremely difficult. Corroborating history from family, friends, or other sources may be important in the ultimate assessment of the patient's condition.

Pharmacology of Pain Control

This section is not meant to be a pharmacological primer for the medical staff. The prescribing physicians should consult primary sources such as the *Physicians' Desk Reference* or pharmacology textbooks before prescribing. It is best to be completely familiar with a few drugs rather than to have a general knowledge of a large number of medications. The information presented in this section is not complete, and is intended only to highlight the important issues concerning the psychological aspects of the burn and trauma patient.

INHALATION AGENTS

Any inhalation anesthesia can be used to control pain, but this approach is rarely used because of the increased risk to the patient. Nitrous oxide is probably the safest of this group of agents and, at times, is used on a temporary basis, since any long-term use would bring with it the risk of bone marrow depression (2).

LOCAL ANESTHESIA

Infiltration with a local anesthetic can be effected prior to the placement of intravenous and intraarterial lines. Local anesthesia is almost always used prior to the insertion of chest tubes and pulmonary arterial catheters. Small doses of narcotics are sometimes used prior to the latter procedures. Narcotics will not only control the pain, but will also provide a sedative effect and help alleviate the anxiety that the patients may have. In such situations, the benzodiazepines are the first choice to control anxiety and produce slight sedation. This class of drugs is frequently used before endoscopy and bronchoscopy. If intravenous lines are in place, narcotics may be administered via this route.

NERVE BLOCKS

Pain control with rib fractures can be achieved by utilizing intercostal nerve blocks, which are long-acting local anesthetics. The techniques will not be discussed here. It is important to note, though, that when numerous ribs are being blocked, or large doses of the nerve blocks are otherwise being used, there can be systemic sedation or toxicity due to inadvertent intravascular injection or overdose. In the same manner, when epidural analgesia (anesthesia) is used in trauma cases or following abdominal thoracic or spinal surgery, the patient must be monitored for any systemic effects.

Decreased respiratory movement caused by pain, especially with thoracic injury, can decrease aeration and compromise clearance of tracheobronchial secretions, leading to atelectasis and pneumonia.

NARCOTIC ANALGESICS AND THEIR EFFECTS

Morphine remains the prototype drug against which other narcotic medications are measured; it is the standard of comparison in the equianalgesic charts (see Table 1.1). Morphine and related opioids produce their major effects on the central nervous system and the bowel. The analgesia occurs without loss of consciousness; but drowsiness, changes in mood, respiratory depression, decreased gastrointestinal motility, nausea, vomiting, and alteration of the endocrine and autonomic nervous systems can occur (1). In individuals who experience euphoria, the effect is increased with higher doses. The analgesic effects are selective; sensory modalities such as touch, vibration, vision, and hearing are not obtunded. Continuous dull pain is relieved more effectively than sharp intermittent pain. However, with sufficient amounts of morphine, it is possible to gain good pain control even with severe secondary degree burns or in cases of multiple trauma. Particularly in burn patients, this titration can lead to very high doses. In our burn unit at Westchester County Medical Center, some patients have been

Table 1.1. A Comparison of Major Analgesics with Respect to Dosage, Duration and Side Effects (Parenteral Use)[a]

Drug	Equianalgesic Doses (mg)	Parenteral: Oral Dose Ratio Total Pain Relief	Duration of Action in Normal Hepatic Function (hours)	Sedation
AGONISTS				
Morphine	10	1:6[b]	4–6	**[c]
Codeine	120–130	1:2	4–6	*
Heroin	5	1:12	4–5	**
Hydromorphone	1.5	—	4–5	*
Levorphanol	2	1:10	4–6	**
Oxymorphone	1–1.5	1:6	4–5	***
Oxycodone (oral)	10–30	1:2	4–6	**
Meperidine	75–100	1:3	2–4	*
Propoxyphene (oral)	60–90	—	2–3	*
Methadone	7.5–10	1:2	3–8	*
AGONIST-ANTAGONISTS				
Pentazocine	45–60	1:3	2–3	** or stimulation
Butorphanol	2	—	3–4	**
Nalbuphine	10	—	3–6	**
Buprenorphine	0.4	—	4–6	**

	Emesis	Respiratory Depression	Constipation	Physical Dependence
AGONISTS				
Morphine	**	***	***	**
Codeine	*	*	* +	*
Heroin	**	?	***	***
Hydromorphone	*	**	*	**
Levorphanol	**	**	?	**
Oxymorphone	***	***	***	***
Oxycodone	**	**	** +	**
Meperidine	**	**	*	**
Propoxyphene	*	*	?	*
Methadone	*	**	*	*
AGONIST-ANTAGONISTS				
Pentazocine	**	**	*	*
Butorphanol	**	***	***	*
Nalbuphine	**	***	***	*
Buprenorphine	**	***	***	*

[a] © 1990 Micromedex Inc.—All rights reserved—Vol. 66 Exp. 11/30/90.
[b] Although single-dose studies established the relative potency of PO/IM morphine as 6:1, in practice, repetitive dosing is the rule, and a ratio of 3:1 is more commonly used. From Principles of analgesic use in the treatment of acute pain and chronic cancer pain. Skokie, IL: American Pain Society, 1989.
[c] Key
 * Least
 ** Moderate
 *** Most
 + Clinical experience does not demonstrate any significant difference between oxycodone and codeine in terms of their constipative side effect.

gradually titrated upward to dosages in the range of 100 to 200 mg/day I.V. (This will be further explained in the pain protocols below.)

Opioids alter the sensation of pain and may elevate the pain threshold. However, opioids also change the affective response as well. When pain does not evoke its usual responses of anxiety, fear, and panic, a patient's ability to tolerate the pain may be markedly increased even when the capacity to perceive this sensation is relatively unaltered (1). This is why we often consider the addition of synergistic medications, such as tranquilizers or tricyclic antidepressive medications, described below.

Sedation

When narcotics such as morphine are instituted, sedation is an immediately expected result. Sometimes there is a very narrow margin between pain relief and sedation. For the patient whose pain has not been well controlled, the immediate increase in sleep from a narcotic may reflect a peaceful rest associated with proper relief, not overmedication. Patients and families should be warned that sedation is to be expected in the initial phase of narcotic dosing, but that the sedation is expected to decrease over the first 48 to 72 hours. Sedation should not be equated with pain relief. Other causes of sedation such as undiagnosed organic pathology or psychological factors such as depression and withdrawal should be considered.

Central Nervous System Effects

The effect of morphine and its derivatives on the central nervous system are well known: weakness, headache, agitation, tremor, uncoordinated muscle movements, seizures, alterations of mood including nervousness, apprehension, depression, floating feelings, dreams, muscle rigidity, transient hallucinations, disorientation, visual disturbances, insomnia, and increased cranial pressure. Sometimes signs and symptoms of delirium will be indistinguishable from a delirium or organic mental syndrome due to another etiology. These issues will be discussed in the chapter "Organic Mental Syndrome." A single therapeutic dose of a morphine-like opioid can produce a change in the EEG with a shift toward increased voltage and lower frequencies (1).

Pupils constrict when morphine is administered in toxic doses. Pinpoint pupils are pathognomonic of this condition. However, marked mydriasis occurs when asphyxia intervenes.

Respiratory Effect

Morphine and morphine-like opioids depress respiration by acting directly on the brainstem respiratory centers. Death from morphine poisoning almost always occurs due to respiratory arrest. Therapeutic doses of morphine depress all phases of respiratory activity, including rate, minute volume, and tidal exchange. While respiratory depression can occur with opioids, pain is an analeptic. Diminished respiratory volume is due primarily to a slow breathing rate. Obviously, if a patient is on a ventilator, these effects can be counteracted by artificial ventilation. By definition, patients who are experiencing pain are not experiencing central respiratory depression. The respiratory rate is not the essential marker of a toxic effect by opioids. Minute volume and blood gas values, along with clinical assessment, are the best methods for measuring toxic effect (5).

One medication that can be a problem for patients on a ventilator is fentanyl, which has been reported to paralyze respiratory muscles (12). In such an emergency situation, a patient could breathe if instructed to do so. It is important to remember that pain is a natural antidote to respiratory depression and that as tolerance to the narcotic develops, so does tolerance to the respiratory depressive effect. As described below, high doses of narcotics can be counteracted in emergency situations by using a narcotic antagonist.

Nausea and Vomiting

When first introduced, a morphine or opioid derivative may cause nausea or vomiting either by delaying gastric emptying or by direct effect on the gastrointestinal tract (13). In such situations, aspiration is always a dangerous possibility, particularly when the patient is sedated with a decreased cough reflex.

The nausea and vomiting produced by morphine are also caused by direct stimulation of the chemoreceptor trigger for emesis in the medulla. Some patients never vomit after morphine; others do so each time they receive the drug. Nausea and vomiting are relatively uncommon in recumbent patients given therapeutic doses of morphine, whereas nausea occurs in 40% and vomiting in 15% of ambulatory patients, suggesting a vestibular etiology to the symptom (1). The emetic effect can sometimes be counteracted by phenothiazine derivatives, such as Compazine (prochlorperazine), 5 mg orally every 4 hours, or the same dose i.m. or in suppository form. If phenothiazine is not sufficient, any type of antiemetic such as Dramamine, 50 mg, can be added to handle these symptoms. In the case of a gastric outlet obstruction, Reglan may be more useful for some patients in doses of 10 mg every 8 hours.

Cardiovascular Effects

In the supine patient, therapeutic doses of morphine or similar opioid derivatives have no major effects on blood pressure or cardiac rate and rhythm. Patients can have orthostatic hypotension and fainting may occur. The ECG is not directly altered by morphine.

Constipation

Morphine and related opioids cause decreased stomach and bowel motility. There is increased tone in the antral portion of the stomach and the first part of the duodenum. The passage through the duodenum of gastric content is delayed for as many as 12 hours, and therefore the absorption of drugs can be hindered. Biliary and pancreatic secretions diminish and the digestion of food in the small intestine is slowed. Peristaltic waves in the colon diminish after morphine, leading to constipation (1).

Constipation is an inevitable problem with the prolonged use of any narcotic administration, and patients have reported that the pain of constipation can be worse than the pain being treated. It is necessary to use a preventive, aggressive, and regular approach in the management of constipation. Senokot is a natural laxative that induces peristalsis, is colon specific, and can be expected to effectively counteract the effects of morphine within 8 to 10 hours. Dosage of 1 to a maximum of 2 teaspoons twice a day, or 1 tablet to a maximum of 4 tablets twice a day, is used for adults. The medication is adjusted as needed. Stool softeners such as Colace, up to 2 tablets three times a day or a combination of Senokot and a stool softener can be used. Pericolace, a mild peristaltic, can also be used. These medications should be started at the same time that the narcotic is begun. Occasionally, bulk laxatives, low enemas, or manual disimpaction may be necessary. It is essential to assess bowel status regularly and to treat accordingly.

Urinary Symptoms

Morphine can augment the tone of the detrusor muscle of the urinary bladder, causing urinary urgency. The tone of the vesical sphincter is also enhanced by morphine, sometimes making urination difficult (1).

Miscellaneous Effects

Morphine can also cause sweating and pruritus through several general mechanisms.

New Drugs

New drugs for the relief of pain are constantly being tested. The use of I.V. Fentanyl and Midazolam for dressing changes in burn patients was reported at the 1989 American Burn Association annual meeting. The study of 256 patients admitted over 2 years to the University of Michigan Burn Center considered this new pain control technique superior to the usual use of morphine. Patients, staff, and physicians unanimously reported positive response. Physical and occupational therapists noted improved compliance with therapy regimes, including ambulation, and an increased level of consciousness during the posttreatment period.

Fentanyl is many times more potent than morphine and has a significantly shorter duration of action. While the slow intravenous administration of the medication must be supervised by anesthesia personnel, this technique has promise for pain control. Fentanyl patches that are applied to the skin and deliver sustained pain relief are also being introduced.

ONSET AND DOSAGE OF PAIN MEDICATION

The time to the onset and the duration of action of any particular pain medication can be influenced by several factors, such as route of administration, lipophilicity, relative rate of association with the opioid receptor, rate of dissociation from the receptor, and drug metabolism (5). Opioid analgesics do not have an effective serum level or therapeutic window that provides analgesia for all patients. It is necessary, therefore, to titrate the response when using these agents if optimal analgesia is to be obtained (5). In general, a long-acting analgesia is useful for continuous pain and a short-acting analgesia is appropriate for acute pain (8).

In the immediate postinjury period, the majority of patients respond to a dose of 10 mg of morphine sulfate, i.m. or I.V. This is a standard dosage that is equivalent to the analgesic dose of meperidine, 75–100 mg, i.m. At times, for a burn patient, a much higher dose must be used. An explanation is given below in the discussion of optimal dosage under "PRN Versus Around-the-Clock Pain Control"; and guidelines are presented in the "Pain Protocols" section below and in the equianalgesic chart (Table 1.1). Morphine and meperidine are particularly useful in acute pain because of their rapid onset of action and short duration.

DRUG ABUSE AND DEPENDENCY

Opioid analgesics such as morphine may cause psychological and physical dependence. Physical dependence results in withdrawal symptoms in patients who abruptly discontinue the drug. Withdrawal symptoms also may be precipitated through the administration of drugs with narcotic antagonistic activity, such as naloxone, or with mixed agonist/antagonist analgesics, such as pentazocine. Physical dependence usually does not occur to a clinically significant degree until after a few weeks of continued narcotic usage or after a shorter period of time with very large doses. Tolerance, in which increasingly large doses are required to produce the same degree of analgesia, is initially manifested by a short duration of analgesic effect and, subsequently, by decreases in the effectiveness of the analgesia.

It is obviously important to gradually reduce the narcotic once the need for pain control ceases. Ideally, this should be done while the patient is in the hospital and over the appropriate amount of time (see Protocol G, Tapering of Narcotic Medications, in the "Pain Protocols" section below).

Patients properly treated for pain during trauma or burn injury do not become addicted or physically or psychologically dependent on the pain medication if it is gradually reduced. We personally know of very few cases where a person without a previous drug problem was addicted to pain medication following appropriate hospital treatment, although this is a common concern among patients and some medical staff (15, 16). In one study of 11,822 patients who received opioids, only 4 were reported to have developed iatrogenic dependency (14).

UNDERMEDICATION FOR PAIN

Despite the fact that pain management is of major concern to the medical and nursing staff and that much time and energy are spent regulating medication to control pain, patients frequently feel that their pain is not adequately controlled. Staff involved with the psychological care of patients also often conclude that patients treated for burn and trauma are frequently undermedicated for pain.

On the surface, several concerns verbalized by medical and nursing staff could account for this phenomenon. As discussed above, it is a common misconception of staff that patients given large amounts of narcotics for pain control are candidates for "addiction" to such medication. Of course, it is true that there can be tolerance and physiological as well as psychological dependence on these drugs during the hospital phase of treatment. But the medications can be gradually reduced and discontinued in such a way that residual physical dependence will not occur. (See pain protocol G.)

It is most important to distinguish between tolerance and physical dependence. Traditional clock-watching is an early sign of drug tolerance or learned pain behavior, not addiction (17). Furthermore, staff may not realize that intramuscular narcotics do not produce a euphoric "rush" (18).

On some occasions, underlying psychological factors may lead to a patient's exaggerated pain response, and these factors should be addressed.

However, especially during the acute phase of burn and trauma treatment, in situations with definitive injuries, there is no doubt about the existence of significant pain. Patients with preexisting emotional problems may have a decreased threshold to pain stimuli; and patients with a history of substance abuse may have increased tolerance to pain medication. However, in these situations, as in any injury, "pain is soul destroying and no patient should have to endure intense pain unnecessarily" (19).

We need to look further for an understanding of undermedication for pain. McMorrow has found that the amount of education that the nurse has had about pain influences the adequacy of pain medication that that nurse gives to patients (20). Perry has a thought-provoking hypothesis concerning the underlying psychological reasons for the persistent undermedication of pain. He suggests that the preservation of pain in the physically ill meets certain unconscious needs for both the caretaker and the patient, and that the staff's unconscious need for pain is not primarily sadistic in nature (15). We entirely agree that the overwhelming majority of staff are often quite upset by the pain inflicted on patients during burn treatment. At times the staff will have symptoms and dreams characteristic of posttraumatic stress.

However, Perry makes the point that the staff often have mixed reactions to the patient's pain. On one hand, they seem to be aware of what patients endure and to feel that they would rather die than undergo this experience. On the other hand, often with the same patient, they contend that the patient does not hurt that much and is merely "overreacting," "anxious," "hysterical," or "malingering" (15). After further study of this issue, Perry defines the unconscious forces contributing to the staff's resistance to using more adequate dosages of analgesic. The patient's pain serves two important functions: it makes the patient a definable being, separate from the staff; and it helps to confirm that the "object" is alive. A pain-free, disfigured burn patient might be experienced as "fading away" or in "the shadow of death" (15).

Perry suggests techniques for handling these issues: Point out differences between the caretaker and the patient and describe the patient as a separate, well-defined individual (mention his or her struggles with adolescent children, the recent purchase of a new home, worries over a failing grandmother . . .). Also, it is useful to describe to the staff some aspects of the patient, other than the pain, that make him animate (or alive), such as his moods, fears, fantasies, appetite, and wish (if not ability) to be mobile. Perry emphasizes that narcotic analgesics do not remove pain, but only make the patient "indifferent" to this sensation, thereby implying that the pain (and the "aliveness") would still be present at higher dosages of medication.

Perry extends his understanding of this unconscious mechanism to include the patient. Based on his observations of patients who used self-regulated analgesics with a special patient-controlled analgesia pump, he observed that the patient chose not to remove all of his pain, but rather to reduce it to tolerable levels. He felt that without some pain patients lose their sense of reality (15). He further notes the problems of patients who are completely immobile because of the use of a paralyzing medication such as Pavulon. These patients may need some sensation to establish their own existence.

In the reality of pain management, all sensations of pain regarding the injury will never be eliminated, although this should be a primary goal of the treatment team. There should be constant reviews of the success in meeting this pain-free goal. Such reviews should include the self-examination of any psychological resistances toward this end. Ultimately, it is the philosophy of the treatment team that will determine the pain control achieved.

NONNARCOTICS

Nonsteroidal Antiinflammatory Drugs

Narcotics relieve pain primarily by attacking the CNS; nonnarcotics relieve pain by attacking the peripheral nervous system. For this reason it is useful to recognize the value of combining a narcotic with a nonnarcotic such as a nonsteroidal antiinflammatory drug (NSAID) or an acetaminophen such as Tylenol. Salicylates (aspirin) can also be useful NSAIDs, especially in the enteric-coated form.

Aspirin is the NSAID of first choice for some because it is the least expensive. However, it is the only NSAID with direct toxic effect on the mucosa of the stomach and an effect on bleeding time—it destroys platelets, which may cause an increase in bleeding time (21). If aspirin is being used for its pain-relieving properties, the employment of other NSAIDs in combination is not recommended. The aspirin will decrease their effectiveness by combining with the same protein-binding sites.

Tylenol has less power as an anti-inflammatory but generally fewer side effects than other NSAIDs, and it may be given with other NSAIDs without decreasing their effect. Tylenol #3 and Tylenol #4 (Tylenol with codeine) contain only 300 mg of Tylenol and can be even more effective when added to another plain Tylenol in order to increase the NSAID property without the increase in codeine, which may be too sedating.

Ibuprofen (Motrin, Advil, and Nuprin) may be better tolerated than aspirin or Tylenol in some patients, and can be useful. This set of NSAIDs was originally introduced and marketed primarily for the treatment of arthritis. Now many of these drugs are also used as general analgesics.

It is virtually impossible to predict which patient will respond to which NSAID. However, it is useful to ask a patient: "What do you take for relief of general pain such as a headache or muscle pain?" Most individuals need to know we recognize that the severity of their pain (as that in burns or multiple fractures) will not be relieved by NSAIDs alone, but that there may be a use for the common pain-relieving drugs in conjunction with narcotics. Examples follow.

CASE STUDY

A 23-year-old man was in the burn center for second and third degree burns over 30% of his total body surface. He required 30 mg of morphine I.V. for wound debridement. Between his two daily dressing changes he had only mild "background" pain, which was relieved by two extra strength Tylenol.

Another patient with the same injury might require around-the-clock morphine or a similar narcotic to control such background pain. Each individual has a different pain experience and a different pain threshold.

CASE STUDY

A 75-year-old woman was hospitalized with multiple fractures from a motor vehicle accident. For pain she was given Percocet, 1 or 2 tablets every 4 hours, PRN. She experienced nausea, vomiting, and dizziness after taking the Percocet.

We learned during an interview with the patient that she usually had relief from headache or similar pain with one-half or 1 Bufferin tablet. It was suggested to the staff that Bufferin be utilized for pain control and this change proved effective in relieving the patient's pain.

Some patients with moderate-to-severe pain may respond to mild analgesics. It is important to obtain a patient's history.

Ketamine

Ketamine is a nonbarbiturate, general anesthetic agent that produces a dissociation in the brain between the thalamic function and the limbic region. It produces a state of inactivity on the part of the patient, who will have no conscious recall of the procedure endured. The eyes may remain open, as if the patient were in a state of catatonia (22).

Low-dose I.V. ketamine (1 to 3 mg/kg body weight) has proved to be useful for shorter treatments—particularly painful debridements, brief operative procedures, or diagnostic procedure—lasting 5 to 30 minutes. A brief scrapping and grafting procedure with ketamine obviates the intubation required for general anesthesia.

Ketamine must be administered by trained personnel only, usually staff of the anesthesiology department. Side effects of ketamine include arterial hypertension, tachycardia, excessive upper airway secretions, and also postoperative psychological reactions of altered mood, dreamlike states, and delirium. These latter effects are of particular interest.

The psychological manifestations of ketamine use vary in severity among pleasant dreamlike states, vivid imagery, hallucinations, and emergent delirium that occurs as the medication wears off. In some, these states have been accompanied by confusion, excitement, and irrational behavior, which a few patients recall as having been unpleasant. The duration is ordinarily no more than a few hours postadministration. No residual psychological effects are known to have resulted from the use of ketamine. It is reported that the emergent dreamlike states and the emergent delirium may be reduced by using lower recommended doses of ketamine in conjunction with an I.V. benzodiazepine such as diazepam. It is also reported that these reactions may be reduced if verbal, tactile, and visual stimulation of the patient is minimized during the recovery period, but this obviously does not preclude the monitoring of vital signs. A severe emergent reaction can be terminated by the use of a small hypnotic dose of a short-acting or ultra-short-acting barbiturate (23).

Antidepressants

Antidepressants, especially in the tricyclics, have been advocated in the treatment of chronic pain. Research has shown that they may be effective and that they work directly on pain perception in doses less than those required for therapeutic antidepressant effect. We have not found this class of drugs useful in the relief of acute pain.

Antidepressant medications may be especially helpful in the treatment of chronic pain when the pain is accompanied by significant depression with vegetative signs, unresponsiveness, persistent sleep difficulties, panic disorder, or persistent unresponsive pruritus. When used for symptoms other than those of depression, doses of antidepressives may be smaller than the doses required for therapeutic levels of antidepressant effect.

Patients who have been taking monoamine oxidase inhibitors during the previous 2 weeks should not be given Demerol (meperidine) because of the risk of severe interactions causing possible fatal hypotension or coma (24).

Tranquilizers

The use of tranquilizers as an adjunct in the treatment of pain is important. Tranquilizers will reduce anxiety and thus raise the pain threshold. Therefore, tranquilizers and narcotics act synergistically. And, when used together, a lesser amount of narcotic may be needed. Tranquilizers should *not* be used as a substitute for pain control.

The benzodiazepines are the most common tranquilizers used as adjuncts to narcotics for pain control in burn and trauma patients. It must be taken into account that this class of medication is synergistic with narcotics in regard to sedation and depressed respiration. Patients receiving narcotics may already be significantly sedated. The patient should never be sedated to the point where he or she cannot be easily aroused. Sometimes the desired clinical situation might be a "twilight state." In rare cases, where the combined use of narcotics and benzodiazepines produces a dangerous state of respiratory depression, a narcotic antagonist such as Narcan can be given. (See Protocol H, below.) This will reverse the action of the narcotic, not the benzodiazepine. However, since the two medications are synergistic with regard to respiratory depression, a relief of the breathing problem should be accomplished. Whenever a narcotic antagonist is utilized to reverse the undesirable effects of respiratory depression, prepare for the possibility of the patient experiencing an upsurge of extreme pain, since the narcotic will not be available for pain control.

PRN VERSUS AROUND-THE-CLOCK PAIN CONTROL

Continuous pain requires continuous analgesia. The aim of any pain relief protocol is to prevent the resurgence of pain rather than to repeatedly treat it. Thus, when ongoing pain is anticipated, around-the-clock dosing rather than PRN is desirable. While PRN narcotic orders must be written for breakthrough pain, the basis of control should be regular scheduling. This strategy maintains the patient's comfort and minimizes negative psychological aspects of pain that may exacerbate the patient's clinical condition and increase the analgesic requirements (5).

With PRN dosing discussed below, patients frequently experience significant pain before they are "eligible" to receive the next dose of the drug. And, if intramuscular doses are used, a drug will not usually become effective before 15 or 20 minutes. Aware that the medication will wear off, the patient often has some anticipatory anxiety, which will also exacerbate the pain. It has been suggested, through clinical experience, that *maintaining* an analgesic will result in less total analgesia being used in 24 hours compared to a method where the pain is "chased" on a PRN basis when it does return.

Patients may decline appropriate doses of analgesics because of fears of dependence or mistaken beliefs that if they take the pain medication when the pain is not severe it will not be effective when they need it later (5).

PRN dosing of pain medication does not recognize the pharmacokinetics of pain medications designed to have a set duration of effect. PRN medications are useful when one expects the pain to diminish rapidly over time, to have a very short duration, or to occur sporadically.

Behaviorally, PRN medicating of pain trains a patient to expect to have to complain, to expect to have to convince a team that the pain is real, and to increase pain behaviors. (How much do I have to cry to convince you that my pain is bad?) At this point the nurses are likely to treat the patient as a stimulus that is noxious to them, believing that the patient is demanding, whining, or acting like a baby. PRN is meant to be as "as needed by the patient," not at the prerogative of the RN (25–27).

When medication orders are written, for example, as 10 mg morphine every 4 hours PRN pain, the nurse is given no authority to assess and treat the patient's pain, and the patient is told that the pain will *only* be treated every 4 hours no matter how much pain is experienced before that time period elapses. An order of morphine 10 mg every 2–4 hours PRN gives some flexibility to cover unanticipated increases in pain *as they occur*. If the demand for pain medication is more frequent than every 2 hours, the dose is obviously not enough, or perhaps a continuous infusion for proper pain control should be considered. (See protocol C.)

PLACEBO

Studies on the effectiveness of placebo in controlling pain vary. Between 20% and 35% of patients have been shown to receive some relief of pain from a placebo. Often patients will have a one-time placebo effect, but no effect afterward.

We feel that there is no place for the use of placebo for pain control in the burn or trauma patient. The placebo effect does not indicate that the pain has a psychological basis or that the patient is exaggerating the pain. In most instances, placebos are used in frustration, when treating demanding or disliked patients or those who do not respond to the standard pain control protocol. Placebo use provides the caregiver with no new information in the treatment of the patient's pain, and opens the door to mistrust and anger which can only aggravate the pain control process.

PATIENT-CONTROLLED ANALGESIA

In support of the idea that the "patient knows best how much pain he or she is experiencing" is the recent development of methods for patient-controlled analgesia (PCA). The PCA pump is a computerized device integrating a small microprocessor with a syringe pump that initiates the injection of analgesia to a patient via an indwelling intravenous catheter. Following an initial bolus injection of medication for pain control, the patient initiates subsequent doses of medication before pain is firmly reestablished. With this program, the patient knows that relief from pain will come and that the drug will be effective. With PCA there is no 15-minute waiting period for the nurse to prepare the injection and administer it; there is no outside party who decides the time for relief. Obviously, the maximum allowable amount of medication over a particular time is established and limited so that the patient does not receive an unsafe dosage.

PCA pumps are not for every patient. There is an initial start-up cost for the pump itself. The equipment must be maintained and the staff educated in its use. The patient must be oriented, able to make judgments, and sufficiently mobile to trigger the pump mechanically. Obviously, a patient with cognitive defects will not be able to operate the apparatus.

A patient who uses the pump may have less interaction and involvement with the staff. The contact time between patient and nurse when medication is administered can be a meaningful, friendly, and gratifying time for the patient.

One study comparing regular dosing with the use of the pump concluded that the difference was not the pump per se, but rather that the patient's severe pain was not allowed to become reestablished (28). The same effect might be obtained with around-the-clock medication. Another study found fault with the pumps because some models failed to accommodate bolus doses of medication that allow a patient to reach an appropriate therapeutic window of pain control when painful procedures are performed (29). It has been suggested that the PCA pump is not more effective than a continuous infusion of pain medication plus supplements (30). PCA pumps are the "new toy on the shelf," but patient-controlled analgesia is far from new. Patients at home on their own may decide which medication and how much should be taken.

Oral PCA could also be utilized in a hospital. In one study, 26 postsurgical patients were given a supply of Tylox to keep at the bedside to self-administer, charting intake on hospital medication sheets. The patients on PCA were able to account accurately for the medications and experienced no overdose, and no greater intake than those given medication by nurses (31).

We believe that analgesia delivered via a patient-controlled pump may be particularly useful for the high-anxiety patient who does not easily establish trust with the staff or who has had a previous negative experience with pain control. For the patient experiencing the frustration of loss of control, PCA may also be a tremendous boost to morale.

Even though further studies using PCA need to be done, the method is useful for the pain control repertoire of any burn or trauma unit.

Guided Imagery and Controlled Relaxation

It is generally accepted and well documented that relaxation enhances the effectiveness of pain medications by reducing muscle tension and increasing blood flow. The use of even simple rhythmic breathing, a back rub, hand or foot massage, hand holding, or touch help a patient relax (32).

Although many patients have their own techniques for relaxation, others can be taught one of a variety of techniques to use as an adjunct to pain medication, an aid in falling asleep, or a pleasant distraction from the tedium of days or weeks in an acute care setting. Slow breathing in through the nose and out through the mouth accompanied by the verbal cue to consciously relax specific muscle groups or body parts can help a person get through a painful procedure.

To individualize a relaxation image for a specific patient, it is useful to ask the patient to describe a favorite place and to give details of the sights, sounds, smells, and feelings associated with that place. The patient can be reminded that when he feels tense and in pain he can go in his imagination to that special place, see himself there, and relax. Patients trained to use such guided imagery can "go to the beach" or "drop the line over the boat and fish" to increase a sense of well-being.

Occasionally, patients have developed relaxation rituals with the use of particular music or even their own taped message from a loved one, minister or rabbi, or favorite person. Children, too, can follow the commands of a trusted person when told to breathe in a specific pattern or to imagine lying on a cloud floating gently over the ground.

Patients who do not like the meditative approach to relaxation or who are very anxious often can use a tense/relax approach to dissipate energy when it is "hard to be still." This approach helps the person to begin to identify the difference between feelings of tension and relaxation. Commands such as the following are given to the patient:

1. Clench the right fist . . . relax.
2. Clench the left fist . . . relax.
3. Wrinkle your forehead . . . relax.
4. Wrinkle your nose and shut your eyes tightly . . . relax.

Muscle groups in this tense/relax approach can be changed. Smaller muscle groups may be used, making the technique last longer. Larger muscle groups can be used, making the technique shorter. A period of 3 to 30 seconds of muscle tension followed by the same period of relaxation should be utilized. Patients may have a preference for starting at the head or feet, and often it is beneficial to omit muscle groups that increase the pain (33).

Sometimes a more structured approach utilizing the hypnotic techniques described below are useful.

Hypnosis for Pain Control

The use of hypnosis with burn patients was described by Crasilneck and associates in 1955 (34). They reported that hypnotic and posthypnotic suggestions were successfully used in burn patients in order to control pain. They also found that this technique can be used to improve hydration and nutrition. Ten years later, Bernstein (35) extended the use of hypnosis to pediatric patients. There are many other reports of the use of hypnosis as an adjunct to pain control in the medical, surgical, and trauma setting (36, 37).

Patients and health professionals have misconceptions about hypnotic intervention. The most common follow (38):

1. The patient may become unconscious when hypnotized. In reality some persons may fall asleep during relaxation induction, but patients do not lose consciousness in a trance.
2. The hypnotist has the power of control. In reality this misconception may originate from entertainers who use hypnosis. The idea is unfounded and untrue. Patients will not follow any suggestion that conflicts with their personal value system. They remain in personal and physical control of themselves.

3. The patient may not wake up. In reality, because patients are not asleep during hypnosis the vast majority of time, this concern is unfounded. However, if patients doze off, they are easily awakened and can awaken on their own whenever desired.
4. Patients who are easily hypnotized are mentally weak. In reality, the contrary is true. Patients who have above-average intelligence, highly developed powers of concentration, and active imaginations are the best hypnotic subjects.

It is not within the scope of this book to teach hypnotic techniques. However, we do believe that there is a role for hypnosis in the medical setting, especially in pain control for trauma and burn patients. We suggest that the interested professional be trained in this modality. A course given regularly at the annual meeting of the American Psychiatric Association is an excellent preparation. We know of other excellent courses taught by responsible persons for general physicians, nurses, social workers, and psychologists.

Hypnosis should be an adjunct to pain medication. It should neither be the first means of pain control offered nor a substitute for adequate pharmacological control of pain. If a patient achieves a level of hypnosis along with successful analgesia, the amounts of narcotic and other agents being used might be reduced. However, if the amounts of pharmacological agents are reduced prematurely, the patient will lose confidence in the hypnotist and in the technique.

The value of the hypnotic technique is especially applicable when there are medical contraindications to adequate narcotic control of pain. In the common situation where fear and anxiety are strong components of pain, hypnosis can be used to complement various psychopharmacological and psychotherapeutic techniques. We have found that hypnosis can rarely be introduced when the patient is experiencing severe, acute pain. In such situations, it may be necessary to utilize high doses of narcotics before the idea of hypnosis can be presented to the patient. Sometimes the patient will ask for an additional approach to control the pain and will be receptive to the idea of hypnosis.

A previous positive experience with hypnosis may be a good indicator for its successful use. The absence of previous experience with hypnosis does not mean it cannot work well in a given individual. Before the possibility of hypnosis is introduced to the patient, it is advisable to evaluate the probability of the patient's hypnotizability by using the following eye roll technique, suggested by Spiegel and Spiegel (39):

The patient is told to look at the examiner on an equal eye level. While holding the head in that position the patient is asked to look up "toward your eyebrows; now toward the top of your head." Then the patient is told to "continue to look upward and close your eyes slowly."

The upgaze, which is scored, is a measure of the amount of sclera relative to the size and shape of the eye between the lower border of the iris and the lower eyelid as the subject is gazing upward. What is measured is the amount of sclera rising from below, not how much of the cornea disappears under the upper eyelid. Scoring is according to Fig. 1.5. Additional points are added if both eyes veer inward, causing an internal squint (Fig. 1.6) (39).

Spiegel and Spiegel suggested additional tests to better predict hypnotizability. We have found that anyone scoring 3 or more is usually a good subject.

If the patient is moderately or highly hypnotizable, the chances of a successful experience with hypnosis are greater. Familiarity with the eye roll technique and eye roll scale allow someone who does not practice hypnosis to nevertheless assess a patient. Therefore, the consultant who does use hypnosis can be called in for those patients with a more predictable experience of success with hypnosis. However, even patients with low-grade hypnotizability as indicated on the eye roll technique can be hypnotized, although the chances for success are less likely.

Those who gain familiarity with hypnotic technique will learn that there are many variations in the approach and induction of hypnosis. Our experience has found that it is not worthwhile to attempt to achieve amnesia for the hypnosis. We tell the patients that we want them to remember the session, so they do not have the sensation of losing control. Sometimes, despite this approach, the patient can have amnesia following a successful hypnotic experience. We also attempt to teach patients auto- or self-hypnosis so that they can put themselves into a hypnotic trance even when the hypnotist is not present. If the staff has been alerted to such a situation, they will be able to inform the patient prior to a scheduled procedure, such as a dressing change. The patient can then utilize this technique on his own. As stated above, we do *not* advise hypnosis as a substitute for the pain control achieved by medication. Even self-hypnosis needs to be reinforced on a regular basis and must be practiced by the patient, often with assistance. Hypnotism is a time-intensive technique for the professional, and that may be one of the reasons it is used infrequently. Sometimes, audio tapes especially made by the hypnotist for the patient may be helpful.

The actual imagery used during a session of hypnotism varies with the techniques of the hypnotist. Some of the images may be quite similar to

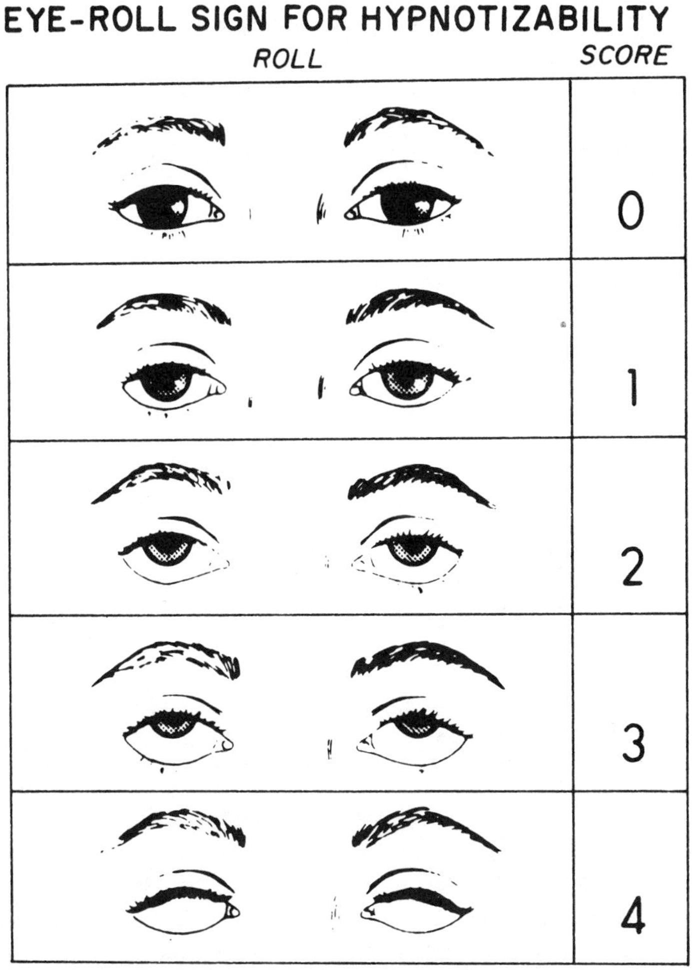

EYE-ROLL SIGN FOR HYPNOTIZABILITY

ROLL   SCORE

Figure 1.5. Eye-Roll Sign for Hypnotizability. Spiegel and Spiegel (39). From Spiegel, H. and Spiegel, D. Trance and Trauma: Clinical Uses of Hypnosis. Copyright © 1978 by Herbert Spiegel, M.D. and David Spiegel, M.D. Reprinted by permission of Basic Books, Inc., Publishers, New York.

those described above under the heading "Guided Imagery and Controlled Relaxation Techniques." For example, during a hypnotic session, the patient may be told that he or she is on a magnificent beach or floating in a beautiful pool or lake. Sometimes an anticipated painful sensation can be transformed into a pleasant one. A patient may be told that he is lying under a waterfall and that the water is cascading pleasurably on his leg. The strong pulsation

EYE-ROLL SIGN (SQUINT) *SCORE*

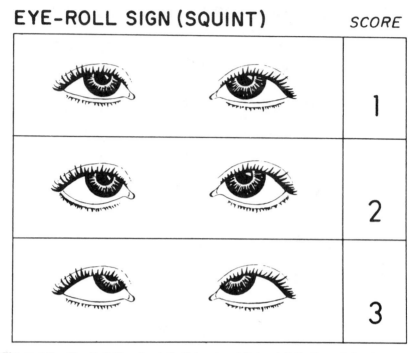

Figure 1.6. Eye-Roll Sign (squint). Spiegel and Spiegel (39). From Spiegel, H. and Spiegel, D. Trance and Trauma: Clinical Uses of Hypnosis. Copyright © 1978 by Herbert Spiegel, M.D. and David Spiegel, M.D. Reprinted by permission of Basic Books, Inc., Publishers, New York.

of the water on an extremity can be associated with an overall happy experience. At the same time, the stimulation of nerve fibers during the dressing change, although recognized, is transformed into a pleasant experience.

We have used hypnosis to achieve complete analgesia during the dressing change of a man with a 35% electrical burn who had experienced unbearable pain even with high levels of narcotic. We have used hypnosis to allow a patient, who could not walk because of unbearable pain, to stroll jauntily around the unit. We have seen many other examples of hypnosis working well as an adjunct to pain control. But we have also tried the hypnotic technique on several patients without success.

Whenever we use hypnosis, we insist on the complete professional demeanor of all staff involved. There is a tendency for people to laugh or joke when hypnosis is discussed or demonstrated. Any suggestion of such behavior on the part of the staff raises the possibility of embarrassment or humiliation for the patient and must be avoided.

A further extension for the use of hypnosis is suggested by Ewin (37, 40–42). He has reported instances where hypnosis was used to prevent the body's inflammatory reaction and believes that the depth and severity of the burn can be attenuated if hypnosis is used early in the course of treatment. We have not used hypnosis in this way, but find these writings quite interesting.

Transcutaneous Electric Nerve Stimulation

Transcutaneous electric nerve stimulation (TENS) has been tried on burn and trauma patients for pain control. TENS is a noninvasive procedure that delivers a mild electric shock to control pain (36). The principle behind TENS involves the gate control theory of pain described above, under the heading "What is Pain?" Analgesia may be produced when cutaneous stimulation interferes electrically with transmission of the pain sensation at the spinal level (43) or when electrical stimulation causes an increase in serotonin, which sensually inhibits the transmission of pain signals (44).

Numerous studies show that although TENS does not work in every patient, there are no real side effects to the treatment (45–48). There may be a problem finding sites for cutaneous application of the impulses in the burn patient due to tissue destruction over a large area of the body.

There are three kinds of TENS: high frequency with low-intensity stimulation, low frequency with high-intensity stimulation (acupuncture), and high frequency with moderate intensity.

A study at the University of Alabama found no statistical differences between TENS and morphine for pain control in a double-blind sample (49). Another study at the same institution showed that 24 patients scheduled for travase enzymatic debridement, a particularly painful procedure, rated TENS as effective as morphine for pain control.

Pain in Children

Before deciding the appropriate way to treat pain in a child, it is necessary to address the general assumptions often made in relation to pain and children. Some believe that the central nervous system of a young child is too immature to experience pain. This notion is used as justification for all sorts of unmedicated procedures. However, in all but the premature infant, the central nervous system is fully mature by 1 month of age (50).

As with adults, there is an erroneous assumption that a certain amount of medication is needed for a set procedure. But children vary as adults do—in expectations, pain tolerance, meaning attached to pain, previous pain experience, and cultural means of expressing pain. Thus, it must be assumed that children's needs for pain medication also vary (51).

The myth that children metabolize opiates differently from adults is simply not supported in the literature. In fact, there is evidence that by 1 month of age children metabolize opiates and excrete the end products as adults do. Morphine is especially effective in children.

Some caregivers would like to believe that young children do not remember painful experiences. This is not at all certain, and may be false.

CASE STUDY

An 18-month-old girl was in the Burn Center for 2 weeks following a hot water scald burn to her legs from overturned soup. At the time of her admission, the child was not yet talking in sentences, and in fact said only a few words. She was especially stoic during burn care and was given little medication because she was "so good."

When the child was a little over 2 years old her mother brought her into the clinic. She was concerned because the child was scraping her doll's legs and saying, "Now don't you cry or I will have to cut off your legs." At the same time, the child was waking at night with terrible dreams. The mother was encouraged to talk with her daughter about the hospitalization and, with use of doll play, was able to correct the child's misconceptions. A coloring book about a dragon who burned his hands when he sneezed was also useful in helping the child work through her burn unit experience.

Issues of addiction and tolerance can be answered in the same way for children as for adults. Caregivers often view children as "too innocent" for the introduction of strong and potentially addicting drugs. There has been no correlation between use of pain medication with injured children and the later development of drug behaviors. As with adults, the caregiver's responsibility to withdraw no longer needed medication by slow tapering should be emphasized.

Dosing of morphine for children can start with the general rule of .1 mg/kg body weight. In general, it is reported that compared to 10 mg morphine, i.m., in adults, children 2 to 6 years of age require one-fifth to one-fourth of that dose. From 7 to 12 years of age, approximately one-half the adult dose is generally effective. Over age 12, most children require the full adult dose, with appropriate weight considerations taken into account (51).

Switching the routes of administration can present the same problems as with adults, sometimes in a more exaggerated way. Children are every bit as capable of knowing the difference in onset of action between intravenous and oral narcotics. They will, like adults, prefer the "fast-acting stuff." To think that this preference is due to abuse or addiction is to fail to recognize the need for education of the child. One way to increase the effectiveness of switching from intramuscular or intravenous morphine to oral administration is to use a combination of both routes, gradually decreasing the intravenous morphine while giving the equivalent increasing dose of oral medication.

CASE STUDY

A 6-year-old child was receiving 5 mg morphine I.V. every 4 hours p.r.n. pain. The following steps were followed to change the routes of administration:

Day 1. Remembering that 1 mg intravenous morphine is equivalent to 3 mg oral (in either pills or liquid form), decrease the q.4 hour intravenous morphine to 3.5 mg and give the remaining 1.5 mg in the oral equivalent of 4.5 mg (1.5 × 3).

Day 2. Decrease the q.4 hour intravenous morphine to 2 mg and additionally give 9 mg orally (3 mg × multiplication factor of 3).

Day 3. Stop intravenous morphine and give 15 mg orally q.4 hours.

In addition to the problem of proper dosing for pain in children, there is the difficulty of dealing with parents. While some parents are insistent that their child not be sedated, others demand that the child be heavily sedated but react frantically when the child shows no open arms and broad grin when Mommy and Daddy arrive to visit.

CASE STUDY

Parents of a 3-year-old boy with several fractures visited with the child for a while and then left the unit. When they returned, their child had received morphine and was very lethargic. "You're killing my baby," was the angry accusation of the mother.

Education is vital, with emphasis on the rationale for proper pain medication and liberal reassurance that as pain decreases, the medications will be withdrawn.

CASE STUDY

Parents of a 6-year-old boy in the Burn Center insisted that every time their child cried he should be medicated for pain. They needed to learn that there were multiple possible reasons for tears (separation, fear, loneliness, to name a few), and that a sedated child cannot fully participate in exercises necessary to prevent contractures or other problems of inactivity.

At times, a compromise may be necessary to accommodate the parents' wishes for their child. When visitation by the family is limited, every effort should be made to time narcotic dosing to maximize parent-child interaction. Alternatively, explaining beforehand that the child will be sleeping and not reacting like him- or herself can go a long way to alleviating the concerns of parents.

A marked difference in pain behavior is often seen in a child when parents are around. This sometimes leads the staff to assume that the child is better off when parents do *not* visit. Such a simplistic conclusion overlooks the following possibilities:

1. Relief of the child at being in the presence of parents, and the freedom to let out contained emotions;
2. A play for sympathy on the part of the child; and
3. An exaggerated concern on the part of the parents that conveys an expectation to the child that the child should be in pain.

Parents can be allies with the staff by telling them what kind of comforting behavior or comfort objects are useful with their child. A careful history from the parents may give clues to how the child normally reacts and whether he or she has had other painful experiences. The particular developmental age of the child will also give clues about managing a painful experience. Can the staff elicit help from the child during painful dressing changes? Can the child be bargained with? ("After you help us with this procedure, we'll go to the playroom.") Perhaps the child is a candidate for guided imagery and the hypnotic techniques previously discussed as adjuncts to medications for pain control.

Additionally, it is important to be alert to individual staff members, who may have particular difficulty handling a child in pain. They may have a child of a similar age. At times they need to vent the feelings that they have been causing pain to a child. A special meeting of the staff may be helpful for sharing feelings in relation to a particular child's pain control problems.

Pain and the Dying Patient

There are times, in the care of trauma or burn patients, when it becomes obvious that the person cannot survive the massive toll of the injury. Then, the goal may be to "just keep the patient free of pain." Certainly, it is important to do that. However, that goal can come long before death is inevitable and when there are still considerations to be addressed in the care of the dying patient.

"If it were me, I would just want to be out of it" is often heard from staff members in regard to a dying patient. In actuality, alert patients who recognize that they are dying often do not want family time to be "missed" by a clouded sensorium. Patients usually know when they are dying (2) and have an agenda to complete. Furthermore, the process of dying may occur without physical pain, but still be psychologically excruciatingly painful, unless compassionate and skilled individuals aid in addressing the issues faced by the dying person and his family. How the end is handled has ramifications for the patient and, especially, for the survivors. Therefore, one would have to carefully titrate the pain medication to allow the patient to have meaningful interaction with his family and at the same time be as free of pain as possible. In such situations, local nerve blocks and regional analgesia may supplement the narcotic medication so that the patient can have a reasonably clear sensorium.

CASE STUDY

A 40-year-old woman with a total body burn and rapidly progressing multisystem failure was seen in our burn unit. She was administered the anesthesia associated with third degree burns, but was alert and aware of her surroundings. She wanted to tell her husband her wishes concerning burial. She was able to hear her husband say "I am sorry for the misunderstandings we have had"; she was able to tell her children once more that she loved them. And they were able to assure her they would take care of each other in the future.

If the patient had been "out of it" with pain medication, she would not have been able to go through this process that was so meaningful to her and to her family.

References

1. Jaffe JH, Martin WR, Opioid analgesics and antagonists. In: Gilman AG, Goodman LS, Rall TW, et al., eds. Goodman and Gilman's The pharmaceutical basis of therapeutics. 7th ed. New York: Macmillan Publishing Co., 1985:491–531.
2. Kram H. Pain management in critically ill trauma and surgical patients. Contemp Surgery 1988; 33(3A)Suppl:26–29.
3. Merskey H, Albe-Fessard D, Benica JJ, et al. Pain terms: recommended by the IASP Subcommittee on taxonomy. Pain 1979;6:249–252.
4. Harrison M, Cotanch PH, Pain: advances and issues in critical care. Nurs Clin North Am 1987;22:691–697.

5. Wolman RL, Lutterman A. Management of pain from burn injury. Contemp Surgery 1988;33(3A)Suppl:20–25.
6. Tempereau C, Grossman RA, Brones M. Psychological regression and marital status: determinants in psychiatric management of burn victims. J Burn Care Rehabil 1987;8:286–291.
7. Tobiasen TM, Hiebert JM. Burn and adjustment to injury. Do psychological coping strategies help? J Trauma 1985;12:1151–1155.
8. Watkins P, Cook L, May R, Ehleben CM. Psychological stages in adaptation following burn injury: a method for facilitating psychological recovery of burn victims. J Burn Care Rehabil 1988;9:376–384.
9. Jensen MP, Karoly R, Braver S. The measurement of clinical pain intensity: a comparison of six methods. Pain 1986;27:117–126.
10. Ohnhaus EE, Adler R. Methodological problems in the measurement of pain: a comparison between the Verbal Rating Scale and the Visual Analogue Scale. Pain 1975;1:379–384.
11. Reading AE. Testing pain mechanisms in pain. In: Wall PD, Melzack R, eds. Textbook of pain. 2nd ed. Edinburgh: Churchill Livingstone, 1989:269–280.
12. Schwab JL. Handbook of psychiatric consultation. New York: Appleton-Century-Crofts, 1968.
13. Levy M. Pain management in advanced cancer. Semin Oncol 1985;12:394–410.
14. Porter J, Jick H. Addiction rare in patients treated with narcotics [Letter]. N Engl J Med 1980;302:123.
15. Perry SW. Undermedication for pain on a burn unit. Gen Hosp Psychiatry 1984;6:308–316.
16. Marks RM, Sachar EJ. Undertreatment of medical inpatients with narcotic analgesics. Ann Intern Med 1973;78:181.
17. Jaffe JH. Drug addiction and drug abuse. In: Gilman AG, Goodman LS, Rall TW, et al., eds. The pharmacological basis of therapeutics. 6th ed. New York: Macmillan Publishing Co., 1980:535–584.
18. Twycross RG. Diseases of the central nervous system: relief of terminal pain. BMJ 1975;4:212–214.
19. Angell M. The quality of mercy. N Engl J Med 1982;306:98–99.
20. McMorrow, MK. Factors affecting the management of burn pain. Unpublished thesis, New York Medical College program in general public health, 1990.
21. McCaffery, M. Pain: Assessment and intervention in nursing practice. In: McCaffery M, ed. Management of the patient with pain. Philadelphia: JB Lippincott, 1972.
22. Gordon MD, Martyn JA, Hondorp M. Ketamine pharmacology and therapeutics. J Burn Care Rehabil 1987;8:146–148.
23. Physicians' desk reference. 44th ed. Oradell, NJ: Medical Economics, 1990, p. 1616.
24. AMA Department of Drugs. AMA drug evaluations 6th ed. Chicago, 1986.
25. Schulte J, Marvin JA, Sandige CH. Can nurses assess patient pain? Fact or fallacy. Presented at the 19th annual meeting of the American Burn Association. Washington, 1987.
26. Iafrati NS. Pain on the burn unit: patient vs. nurse perception. J Burn Care Rehabil 1986;7:413–416.
27. Walkenstein MD. Comparison of burned patient's perception of pain with nurses' perception of patient's pain. J Burn Care Rehabil 1982;3:233–236.
28. Wolman R, Lasecki M, Alexander L, et al. Clinical trials of patient controlled analgesia in burn patients. American Burn Association. Washington: 1987.
29. Woolf CJ, Mitchel D, Barrett GD. Antinociceptive effect of peripheral segmental electrical stimulation in the rat. Pain 1980;8:237–252.
30. Brown L, Creswell S. Patient-controlled analgesia: A state of the art evaluation. Hosp Pharm 1988:144–146.
31. Jones L. Patient-controlled oral anesthesia. Orthop Nurs 1987;6:38–41.
32. Malt RA, McKhahn CF. Replantation of severed arms. JAMA 1964;189:716.
33. McCaffery M. Relieving pain with noninvasive techniques. Nurs 1980;80:55–57.
34. Crasilneck HB, Stirman JA, Wilson BJ, McCranie EJ, Fogelman MJ. Use of hypnosis in the management of patients with burns. JAMA 1955;158:103–106.
35. Bernstein NR. Observations on the use of hypnosis with burned children on a pediatric ward. Int J Clin Exp Hypn 1965;13:1–10.
36. Hilgard ER, Hilgard JR. Hypnosis in the relief of pain. Los Altos, California: William Kaufmann Inc., 1975.

37. Ewin DW. Hypnosis in surgery and anesthesia. In: Wester WC II, Smith AH Jr, eds. Clinical hypnosis: a multidisciplinary approach. Philadelphia: J.B. Lippincott Co., 1984.
38. Chandler C. Hypnoanesthesia and analgesia. J Am Assoc Nurse Anesthetists 1980;38:241–245.
39. Spiegel H, Spiegel D. Trance and trauma: clinical use of hypnosis. New York: Basic Books, 1978.
40. Ewin DM. Clinical use of hypnosis for attenuation of burn depth. In: Frankel F, Zamansky HS. Hypnosis at the Bicentennial. New York: Plenum Press, 1978.
41. Ewin DM. Emergency room hypnosis for the burned patient. Am J Clin Hypn 1983;26:5–8.
42. Ewin DM. Hypnosis in burn therapy. In: Burrows GD, Collison E, Dennerstein L, eds. Hypnosis. Amsterdam-New York: Elsevier/North Holland Press, 1979.
43. Melzack R, Wall PD. Pain mechanisms: a new theory. Science 1965;150:971–979.
44. Woolf CJ, Mitchell D, Barrett GD. Antinociceptive effect of peripheral segmental electrical stimulation in the rat. Pain 1980;8:237–252.
45. Shealy CN, Maurer D. Transcutaneous nerve stimulation for control of pain. Surg Neurol 1974;2:45–47.
46. Cooperman AM, Hall B, Mikalacki K, et al. Use of transcutaneous electrical stimulation in control of postoperative pain—results of a prospective, randomized, controlled study. Am J Surg 1977;133:185–187.
47. Ali JA, Yaffee CS, Serretti C. The effect of transcutaneous nerve stimulation on postoperative pain and pulmonary function. Surgery 1981;89:507–512.
48. Pike, PMH. Transcutaneous electrical stimulation: its use in management of postoperative pain. Anaesthesia 1978;33:165–171.
49. Schafer DW. Hypnosis use in a burn unit. Int J Clin Exp Hypn 1975;23:1–14.
50. Beyer JE, Levin CR. Issues and advances in pain control in children. Nurs Clin North Am 1987;22:661–676.
51. Schechter N, Allen D, Hanson K. Status of pediatric pain control: a comparison of hospital analgesic usage in children and adults. Pediatrics 1986;77:11–15.

PAIN PROTOCOLS

A systematic plan for proper dosage and titration of medication is needed to attack the problem of pain control. This plan must be understood by the physicians who write the orders and the nursing staff who carry them out. It is also essential that the psychosocial team understand this plan. Often, they will be the persons who have prolonged interaction and discussions with the patient about pain control. The dosage of pain medication prescribed by physicians is often inconsistent and ambiguous. The appropriate dosage to administer is often not made clear to nurses. When choices of dosage are allowed, there is the likelihood of inconsistency from nurse to nurse, as well as among the various shifts of staff.

We have developed a set of pain protocols for the administration of pain medication under various circumstances. Our medical and nursing staffs have found this approach to be extremely helpful as a guideline in the administration of narcotics for pain control. Individual treatment teams may change the protocols depending on preference and experience.

We believe, however, that a consistent approach to the management of pain is of distinct value as a starting point for the doctors, nurses, and patients working together. Individual circumstances may require specific changes. But each physician and each nurse has a professional responsibility to understand the clinical situation of the patient and to become familiar with any medications used to treat pain.

Pain Management Protocols

GENERAL PRINCIPLES

1. Pain is whatever the patient says it is when he or she says it. In other words, the patient is the authority on his or her own experience.

2. Patients have a right to pain management that will minimize their physical and psychological suffering.

3. The responsibility for pain control is shared between the patient and the staff and both must be aware of their respective responsibilities.

4. Pain management must be addressed before other psychological issues are addressed.

5. Treatment of pain always involves a three-step process:
   — Assessment (site, nature, intensity, and quality of the pain)
   — Intervention
   — Evaluation (effectiveness of the intervention)

6. Tapering of pain medications is part of the treatment plan.

7. Bowel regimens and pain medications should always be considered simultaneously.

8. Although morphine is used as the drug of choice in the first five protocols to follow, other drugs can be used in the same way. (See "When and how to switch" below.) Morphine has the advantages of wide tolerance and availability in a variety of forms (oral, I.V., i.m. and long-acting slow-release as well as in suppository and liquid forms.

WHEN AND HOW TO SWITCH FROM SUGGESTED MEDICATIONS IN THE
PROTOCOLS TO OTHER MEDICATIONS

1. If the patient has a known or suspected allergy to morphine or to one of
   the other suggested drugs, see the equianalgesia chart for alternative
   medications to use (Table 1.1).

2. If the medication does not relieve pain adequately, do not assume that
   the wrong medication is being used, but consider one or more of the
   following:
   — Increase the dosage.
   — Administer a breakthrough dosage and then increase the regular dosage starting at the next regular interval.
   — Double the next dose at the same interval and evaluate effectiveness
   of new dose.
   — Check to insure that the frequency of the medication is close to the
   analgesic duration for that drug. It may be necessary to decrease the
   interval between doses (increase frequency).
   — Make sure that the medication has been tried on an around-the-clock
   basis as opposed to p.r.n.
   — Remember that dosage of medications can be increased until the
   patient shows negative side effects or toxicity.

3. ONLY in the case of adverse reaction, allergic reaction, or continued
   ineffective relief of pain after the suggestions above have been tried
   would a different medication on the equianalgesia chart be necessary.

Pain Protocols

A. INITIAL TREATMENT OF SEVERE PAIN WITH I.V. MORPHINE—THE FIRST 24 HOURS OF TREATMENT

B. ONGOING TREATMENT OF SEVERE PAIN WITH I.V. MORPHINE

C. TREATMENT OF SEVERE PAIN WITH CONTINUOUS I.V. INFUSION OF MORPHINE

D. TREATMENT OF ONGOING MODERATE TO SEVERE PAIN WITH ORAL MORPHINE

E. LONG-ACTING SLOW-RELEASE ORAL MORPHINE (MS CONTIN) FOR ONGOING MODERATE TO SEVERE PAIN

F. NONMORPHINE ORAL MEDICATIONS FOR TREATMENT OF MILD TO MODERATE PAIN

G. TAPERING OF NARCOTIC MEDICATIONS

H. NARCAN FOR REVERSAL OF THE RESPIRATORY EFFECTS OF MORPHINE

I. BOWEL REGIMENS FOR PATIENTS ON NARCOTICS

Pain Protocols

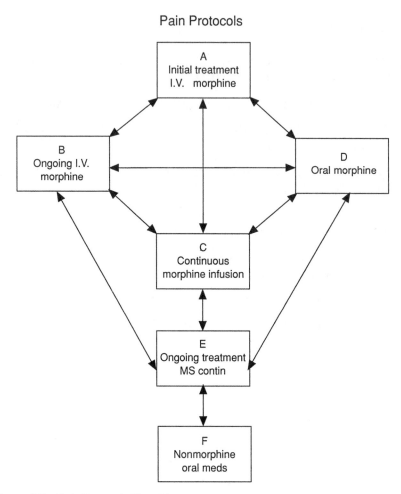

Figure 1.7. Pain Protocols Flow Chart

A. INITIAL TREATMENT OF SEVERE PAIN WITH I.V. MORPHINE—THE FIRST 24 HOURS OF TREATMENT

1. Establish I.V. access.
2. Have Narcan at the bedside (See Protocol H).
3. Administer 10 mg (see * below) I.V. morphine slow push over 1 to 2 minutes.

* This is a general guideline for dosage of morphine in a person aged 12 to 65 years with an average body weight. Circumstances may require higher or lower starting doses. In patients weighing less than 30 kg, use the formula of 0.1 mg/kg body weight in calculating dosage.

C A U T I O N

Administration of morphine should be held if any of the following are noted:
A. Respirations decrease below 10/min.
B. Patient is not easily arousable or is oversedated.
C. Patient is increasingly disoriented and not easily re-oriented.
D. Patient has significant nausea, vomiting, or abdominal distension.
E. Patient's blood pressure drops.
F. Any allergic reaction occurs.

---

4. In 30 minutes evaluate patient's pain control and repeat ½ the initial dose of I.V. morphine if the patient has not shown significant improvement in pain control.
5. If the patient does not have good pain control after 1 hour from initial dosing with morphine, repeat initial dosage of I.V. morphine after making sure that conditions in "caution" above are not present.
6. If pain is still present, repeat initial dose of morphine every 4 hours over the first 24 hours with the following considerations:
   A. In case of breakthrough pain, ½ the dose scheduled for q 4 h may be given at the 2 hour interval, followed by the regular dose 2 hours later.
   B. If the patient requires more than three doses of I.V. morphine in a 6 hour period, he or she may be a candidate for continuous I.V. infusion (see Protocol C.)
7. See Bowel Protocol I for patients on narcotics.

B. ONGOING TREATMENT OF SEVERE PAIN WITH I.V. MORPHINE

1. After 24 hours on I.V. morphine, add up the patient's total 24-hour utilization of I.V. morphine (excluding additional amounts used for special procedures). Divide the total by 8, then give that amount q 3 h around the clock on day two.

CAUTION

Administration of morphine should be held if any of the following are noted:

A. Respirations decrease below 10/min.
B. Patient is not easily arousable or is oversedated.
C. Patient is increasingly disoriented and not easily re-oriented.
D. Patient has significant nausea, vomiting, or abdominal distension.
E. Patient's blood pressure drops.
F. Any allergic reaction occurs.

---

2. If at any time the dosage scheduled for q 3 h does not provide the patient with adequate comfort, one breakthrough dose of ½ the scheduled q 3 h dose may be given.
3. If the patient requires more than three doses I.V. morphine in any six-hour period, he or she may be a candidate for a continuous I.V. infusion of morphine. (See Protocol C.)
4. If at any time the patient establishes bowel sounds and can take medication orally (or in liquid via a nasogastric tube), consider converting the I.V. dose of morphine to oral morphine using Protocol D or E.
5. After every 24 hours, the dosage given q 3 h needs to be recalculated by looking at the total 24-hour requirement and dividing again by 8.
6. If the patient has had good pain control over a 24-hour period, consider tapering the around-the-clock dose by approximately 25% (See also Protocol G for tapering narcotics.)
   Example: A patient receiving 8 mg I.V. morphine q 3 h around the clock reports good pain control for 24 h

   The next day, assuming no anticipated increase in the amount of pain, try 6 mg I.V. morphine q 3 h around the clock.
7. See Bowel Protocol I for patients on narcotics.

C. TREATMENT OF SEVERE PAIN WITH CONTINUOUS I.V. INFUSION OF MORPHINE

Consider continuous I.V. infusion of morphine for the patient who is experiencing moderate to severe pain that after an adequate trial of intermittent or around-the-clock morphine (oral or I.V.) requires dosing at intervals less than q 2 h.

1. Have Narcan at the bedside (see Protocol H).
2. Convert the daily morphine requirement to an I.V. equivalent (oral total divided by 3 equals the I.V. equivalent), and divide the total by 24 to determine the required hourly dose.
3. Mix the calculated morphine dose in I.V. fluid as follows:
   A. For patients receiving 5 mg/h, mix 50 mg of morphine in 250 cc of D5W or NS to yield a concentration of 0.2 mg/cc.
   B. For patients receiving 6 to 10 mg/h, mix 100 mg morphine in 500 cc D5W or NS to yield a concentration of 0.2 mg/cc.
   C. For patients receiving 11 to 30 mg/h, mix 250 mg of morphine in 500 cc D5W or NS to yield a concentration of 0.5 mg/cc.
   D. For patients receiving over 30 mg/h, mix 500 mg of morphine in 500 cc D5W or NS to yield a concentration of 1 mg/cc.
   The previously required daily amount of morphine will now be administered using the appropriate concentrated amounts above delivered at the calculated rate of cc/h.
4. Always use an infusion control device to prevent inadvertent rapid infusion.

C A U T I O N

Administration of morphine should be held if any of the following are noted:
A. Respirations decrease below 10/min.
B. Patient is not easily arousable or is oversedated.
C. Patient is increasingly disoriented and not easily re-oriented.
D. Patient has significant nausea, vomiting, or abdominal distension.
E. Patient's blood pressure drops.
F. Any allergic reaction occurs.

---

5. At infusion initiation and when increasing the infusion rate, begin by administering loading doses as follows:
   A. To maintain a rate of up to 15 mg/h, give 15 mg morphine I.V. push over 2 min.

    B. To maintain a rate of 15–30 mg/h, give 15 mg morphine I.V. push over 2 min.

    C. To maintain a rate of over 30 mg/h, give 30 mg morphine I.V. push over 2 min.

6. At least every 24 hours, recalculate the patient's need for continuous morphine and titrate upward or downward according to the appropriate protocol.

7. When the patient has good pain control, consider tapering the dose by 25%. (See Protocol G.)

8. See Bowel Protocol for patients on narcotics.

D. TREATMENT OF ONGOING MODERATE TO SEVERE PAIN WITH ORAL MORPHINE

CRITERIA FOR SWITCHING I.V. MORPHINE TO ORAL MORPHINE

* Patient is no longer NPO
* Patient has normal bowel sounds
* Surgery is not anticipated for at least the next 24 hours

C A U T I O N

Any administration of morphine should be held if any of the following are noted:
A. Respirations decrease below 10/min.
B. Patient is not easily arousable or is oversedated.
C. Patient is increasingly disoriented and not easily re-oriented.
D. Patient has significant nausea, vomiting, or abdominal distension.
E. Patient's blood pressure drops.
F. Any allergic reaction occurs.

---

1. Make the change from I.V. to oral morphine gradually, as follows:
   Take ½ the I.V. dose of morphine times 3 (the conversion factor for changing I.V. to oral morphine) and give orally. Give the remainder I.V.
   Example: If 10 mg I.V. morphine is given q 3 h, give 15 mg orally (in tabs or elixir) and 5 mg I.V.
   At the next scheduled dosage of q 3 h regimen, give ¼ of the usual I.V. dose and give the remaining ¾ orally.
   Example: If 10 mg I.V. morphine is given q 3 h then give 2 mg I.V. with 20 mg oral morphine.
   At the next scheduled dosage of the q 3 h regimen, give the total usual I.V. dose in its oral equivalent (I.V. dose $\times$ 3 = oral equivalent).
   Example: If 10 mg I.V. morphine is due, then give 30 mg oral morphine.
2. Explain to the patient the following reasons for changing to oral medication from I.V. medication:
   * longer-acting, sustained pain relief
   * fewer peaks and valleys in pain control
   * less likelihood of dependency and increasing tolerance to the medication
3. Teach the patient to expect the following:
   * lack of any "rush" or immediate pain relief with an accompanying feeling of warmth

* longer-acting pain relief over 3 to 4 hours without the need for repeat dosing and with good pain control
4. After 24 hours of good pain control on oral morphine consider tapering the dosage by 25%. (See Protocol G)
5. Patients may also be switched directly to long-acting slow-release morphine (see Protocol E) from I.V. morphine.
6. See Bowel Protocol I for patients on narcotics.

E. LONG-ACTING SLOW-RELEASE ORAL MORPHINE (MS CONTIN) FOR ONGOING MODERATE TO SEVERE PAIN

Consider a patient for long-acting slow-release morphine when all of the following criteria have been met:
* Patient has been tolerating regular morphine well.
* Patient is no longer NPO and can swallow whole pills. (MS Contin tablets may not be crushed or broken due to their slow-release properties.)
* Patient will require ongoing pain relief for moderate to severe pain for at least three days.
* Patient is already taking at least 60 mg/day oral morphine or 20 mg/day I.V. morphine (or its equivalent).

If the above criteria are met, proceed as follows:
1. Determine the amount of I.V. or oral morphine given in the past 24 hours (excluding amounts for special procedures).
2. Convert I.V. morphine to oral equivalent by multiplying by the conversion factor of 3.
3. Now that you have figured the oral dosage needed for 24 hours, take this number and divide by 2 to determine dose of MS Contin to be given q 12 h.

C A U T I O N

    Administration of morphine should be held if any of the following are noted:
A. Respirations decrease below 10/min.
B. Patient is not easily arousable or is oversedated.
C. Patient is increasingly disoriented and not easily re-oriented.
D. Patient has significant nausea, vomiting, or abdominal distension.
E. Patient's blood pressure drops.
F. Any allergic reaction occurs.

---

4. MS Contin is available in 15, 30, 60, and 100 mg tablets and the fewest number of tablets (without exceeding the patient's 24-hour required dose) should be utilized.

    Example #1: If a patient has received a total of 120 mg of oral short-acting morphine (excluding extra amounts for special procedures) in the last 24 hours, then give 120 mg divided by 2 (60 mg MS Contin q 12 h)

Example #2: If a patient has received 70 mg of I.V. morphine in the last 24 hours then give 70 × 3 (210 mg oral morphine q 24 h)

210 mg would mean 105 mg MS Contin q 12 h

To dispense 105 mg MS Contin q 12 h an odd number of MS Contin tablets would be needed if only 30 mg tablets were available. Consider 90 mg in the a.m. and 120 mg at night (or vice-versa, depending on when the patient experiences more pain).

Example #3: If a patient has received a total of 160 mg of oral morphine elixir in the last 24 hours then give 160 mg divided by 2 (80 mg q 12 hours)

Give 75 mg MS Contin q 12 hours (round down to give 75 rather than up to 90 mg).

5. Provide I.V. morphine or oral short-acting morphine for breakthrough pain (10 mg I.V. or 30 mg oral).
6. Every 24 hours, recalculate the MS Contin dosage required. One may need to titrate upward if there was breakthrough pain or downward if tapering is indicated. Rare patients may benefit from q 8 h dosing rather than q 12 h.
7. Tapering of MS Contin can be accomplished by decreasing the dosage by one tablet a day. When the dosage is down to one tablet, it is usually given at night. (See also Protocol G for tapering narcotics.)
8. See Bowel Protocol I for patients on narcotics.

F. NONMORPHINE ORAL MEDICATIONS FOR TREATMENT OF MILD TO MODERATE PAIN

Medication may be initiated by giving

1. Percocet 1 or 2 tablets q 3–4 h p.r.n. pain.

   or

   Tylenol #3 1 or 2 tablets q 3–4 h p.r.n. pain.
2. Use p.r.n. medications when the level of pain is likely to vary with patient activity—i.e., when he or she goes for physical therapy or late in the day when the patient is tired.
3. Use 2 tablets of the above medications when the patient is coming off morphine or other strong narcotics. Consider one tablet when the patient is elderly or has a known sensitivity to pain medications.
4. Hold the medications if any of the CAUTION conditions found in Protocol A, B, C, D, or E exist.
5. Consider switching to around-the-clock dosing if the patient requires at least 10 tablets in a 24-hour period.
6. There are times when a patient on this Protocol will need to be moved to a morphine protocol such as Protocol A, B, C, D, or E due to increased pain.
7. After 24 hours of improved pain control (without medication) or with decreased requests for prn medications, consider switching to regular Tylenol or a nonsteroidal anti-inflammatory such as aspirin or Motrin.
8. See Bowel Protocol I for patients on narcotics.

G. TAPERING OF NARCOTIC MEDICATIONS

When there is a decreased need for narcotics, the medications should be tapered gradually. Although rapid tapering can often be tolerated by a patient, a reduction by ¼ of the total narcotic intake every other day is recommended to decrease the chances that the patient will experience the following disturbing symptoms or a recurrence of pain.

Symptoms of withdrawal:

* tremors
* agitation and increased emotional lability
* rhinorhea
* sweating
* restlessness or sleeplessness

Unless there is a pressing reason for a more rapid withdrawal, if evidence of withdrawal occurs, the rate of withdrawal should be reduced only 10 to 15% q day.

If there is an increase in pain, the previous dosage of pain medication, which controlled the pain, should be reinstated.

Although pain medications should be reduced gradually, there may be times when full tapering of narcotics can not be accomplished before the patient goes home. In this case, a few tablets may need to go home with the patient, along with instructions for continued tapering.

Ideally, the pain medication that the patient will be discharged with is the same as that used over the last 24 hours of inpatient stay.

H. NARCAN FOR REVERSAL OF THE RESPIRATORY EFFECTS OF MORPHINE

Narcan (naloxone) is a useful narcotic antagonist that can be used as follows for the reversal of the effects of opioids, including respiratory depression, sedation, and hypotension.

Administer:

Adults   0.4 to 2 mg Narcan I.V. every 2 to 3 minutes as needed to a maximum of 10 mg.

Children   0.01 mg/kg body weight up to 0.1 mg/kg body weight

The effects of the narcotic antagonist may wear off before the effects of the narcotic. Therefore, the Narcan may need to be repeated, and the patient must be carefully monitored.

The pain relief effect is also likely to be reversed for a patient given Narcan. Therefore, the patient will require reassurance, a reduced dosage schedule, and an alternative medication or pain control approach as soon as possible.

I. BOWEL REGIMENS FOR PATIENTS ON NARCOTICS

Because of the constipating effects of all narcotics, consider putting all patients on a prophylactic bowel regimen and progressing the patient from regimen 1 to 2 and 3, below, as the problem is encountered or an increasing severity is anticipated.

* Assess the patient's normal bowel pattern to determine the desired goal.
  — Does the patient have a bowel movement usually every day, every other day, or several times a day?
  — What is the normal consistency of the movements?
  — Does the patient normally depend on laxatives, and, if so, what does he normally use?
* Educate the patient about the constipating effects of narcotics so that he or she will be aware of the importance of preventing and reporting problems.
* Make certain that the patient is well hydrated and is ingesting adequate amounts of fruits and vegetables, if able to be on a regular diet.
* Provide an opportunity for the patient to use the bedpan, commode, or bathroom without interruptions at least once daily. After breakfast is often the most effective time, but patients vary in their patterns.
* Add one or more of the following to the patient's medication regimens:

  #1. Colace 1 or 2 capsules 2 to 3 times per day
  If loose or frequent stool develops, check first for an impaction and then lower the amount of medication or use #2 below.

  #2. Switch Colace to Pericolace (which contains an added stimulant) 2 to 3 times per day.
  Consider the alternatives of Milk of Magnesia 30 cc, a dulcolax suppository, or a Fleet enema as needed.
  If loose or frequent stool develops, check first for an impaction, and then lower the amount of medication, go back to #1, or start #3 after an impaction has been removed manually or with enemas until clear.

  #3. Give 1 Senokot-S tablet for every 30 mg of MS Contin (contains senna concentrate) or up to a maximum of 8 Senokot-S tablets per day (4 tablets b.i.d.) for a more-difficult-to-manage problem with constipation.

If efforts to prevent constipation are unsuccessful, other medical problems contributing to GI difficulties must be ruled out.

As the narcotics are tapered, the need for a bowel regime is likely to be eliminated as long as the patient can begin normal eating patterns and activity.

Patients sent home on pain medications need to be warned of the possible constipating effects of the drugs.

2

Emergency Room Care of the Patient and Family

The next time you are in your hospital emergency room at a busy time, try this exercise. Imagine you have no medical sophistication. Absorb all the sights and sounds and smells. Look closely at the monitoring equipment, I.V. pumps, bandages, oxygen masks, and tubes. Listen to the words around you: "This one goes to neuro. . . ." "I have a GI bleed in room 6." "You can take a break after you close that laceration." "Room 2 needs to be bagged." Take in the tearful family, the crying child, the paradox of frantic staff members who may be handling a delicate situation with a laid-back demeanor, or someone else who may be wearing a white lab coat but nonchalantly reading a newspaper while a doctor and nurse handle a life and death situation.

An ER is associated with every trauma case, and it is where the patient will first be evaluated. The psychological care of the patient and family ideally begins in this setting.

Psychological Support for the Patient and Family

Trauma usually involves blood and pain and it is difficult, in this setting, to deny the presence of injury. Patients therefore frequently fear the worst. The initial fear of death is paramount for both the patient and the family in any case of serious trauma or burn. Liberal reassurance is needed because the patients cannot themselves evaluate the severity of their injuries. Even when assured, they will later acknowledge that they were sure they were going to die and that no one would tell them the truth.

Family members may have seen their loved one in flames or in a catastrophic accident and be convinced that death is inevitable because nothing so horrible had ever happened or even been imagined before. On the other hand, the patient and his or her family may have an unrealistic expectation associated with the victim's early ability to talk or initial lucidity and calm, rational behavior. Some important initial aspects of support for the patient and family follow:

1. *Give realistic information directly to the patient and family as it becomes available.* This information needs to be short and to the point ("We don't yet know the full extent of the injuries but we are evaluating" or "Try to stay as calm as you can and we will let you know everything we know as we go along.") All possibilities do not need to be initially discussed.
2. *Provide an opportunity for the patient and family to see each other as soon as possible.* This does not need to be a long encounter. The actual visiting with or viewing of loved ones does much to clarify the situation to family members. In some cases it reassures the family, and in others it begins to prepare them for the necessary "worry time." Telling the family beforehand what they will see in the ER is necessary and should be specific. "There will be blood on his head" or "There will be a tube in her nose or her mouth" are important details. No knowledge of medical situations should be assumed. Even when persons have such knowledge, the medical facts may totally escape them at this time.
3. *Be alert to clues of psychological risk factors for both the patient and the family.* There are at least two psychological issues that have to be addressed: the psychological reaction to the trauma itself, and any psychological problem that already existed at the time of the accident (1). The latter will not always be present or apparent, but information about what was occurring, psychologically, for the patient and his or her family at the time of the trauma may be key in the patient's overall psychological recovery or survival. Accidents often happen at the "worst time." In one study, 40% of trauma patients were experiencing severe psychological stress at the time of the trauma (1).

Telling the Patient That Survival Is Not Expected

Sometimes, it may be immediately determined that the patient has an injury for which survival is unprecedented, or, because of a preexisting terminal illness, the usually aggressive ER techniques will not be used.

In such situations, the team caring for the patient may wish to answer the patient's questions about the expected death in an honest and straightforward manner. The decision to explain the patient's condition to him or her will usually be made after consultation with the family and/or with the patient's physician, who may be familiar with the patient's previous wishes. In such a situation, the patient should be reassured that all efforts to eliminate pain will be taken. Obviously, this patient should not be abandoned. Pain control and relief of discomfort should be aggressively continued. This patient should be allowed to have frequent or continuous contact with family and clergy if desired.

It is unusual for a "Do Not Resuscitate Order" or a nonaggressive treatment approach to be utilized in the ER. For the medical staff to be comfortable with this option under certain circumstances, there should be prior staff discussion so that everyone is familiar with the circumstances under which this option will be utilized.

About 13 years ago, Imbus and Zawacki suggested an approach to the burn patient who has a burn from which survival is unprecedented (2). They noted that during the first few hours after a burn injury, even the most severely burned patient was usually alert and mentally competent. When burns were so severe that survival was unprecedented, they used an aggressive approach to decision making, which they believed would preserve patient autonomy. In response to the frequently asked question "Am I going to die?", they would answer truthfully: "We cannot predict the future; we can only say that, to our knowledge, no one of your age and with your burn size has ever survived this injury, with or without maximum treatment." While still lucid and after being given sufficient information, the patient would then be asked to choose between the full therapeutic regime or ordinary care, and receive reassurance that, with either choice, the burn team would provide constant human caring and put its professional skills fully at his or her service.

We have found that this approach is usually *not* compatible with the philosophy of a modern-day ER. Current techniques now make possible the stabilization of patients who frequently would have died in the ER in the past. It seems that any decisions for withdrawing life support will usually be made outside the emergency setting over the next several days. Although at that point the patient may not be able to participate in decisions because of a clouded sensorium or coma, the family will be involved and will be asked to represent the patient's views. However, there may be value in utilizing the technique of Imbus and Zawacki in selected, unique clinical situations.

At the 1990 annual meeting of the American Burn Association, Gillon Ward gave a presentation titled, "The die is cast—telling patients they are going to die." Ward reported on 39 patients, admitted over a 10-year-period, who had what are considered lethal injuries. Of the 39, 15 (38%) were told they were going to die and the other 24 (62%) were not told. Those informed were awake, able to make plans with their families and to say their "goodbyes."

Certainly, there is a precedent for telling patients their prognoses. Surgeons have long operated, found lethal problems, and then told their patients that they were going to die. While we would never suggest that the decision about what to tell the patient is easy, we do believe that each situation needs careful consideration. ER personnel need to have regular dialogues about such issues.

Telling the Family That Survival Is Not Expected

In many ER situations, the job of the staff is to tell a family of the death or imminent death of a loved one. It may be useful for the family to be told in stages. First, the family might be told that things look "very bad" and that supportive and/or significant family members should be called to come to the hospital. A short time later, the family might be told that the patient is even less stable. Then, at the time of death, the family can be told that despite all efforts, the patient has died. This "staging" can give the family a little time to gather its coping reserves.

There are no "good" ways to break the news of the death of a loved one, although there are approaches that are more effective than others in fostering trust and giving support to the family. Some principles that we have found to be useful follow.

1. Have at least two persons from the medical team approach the family in the hospital. The team approach offers advantages for both the family and the caretakers. For the family, an additional person can immediately validate news coming from the spokesperson. If one family member needs to leave the room or becomes very upset, a professional can direct attention to that family member while the other professional is with the rest of the family. A family member may feel faint and in need of immediate assistance.

   For the caretaker, the presence of at least one additional person is a source of emotional support and provides him or her with someone with whom to process the experience afterward. Nurses, doctors, the clergy, mental health professionals, nursing supervisors, and social workers are all potential team members who can be involved in this process. Ideally, one member of the team will be able to stay with the family for a period following the news of the death of a loved one. In fact, the news should usually not be given until such a support can be provided.

2. Refrain from telling family members *how* they should feel. There is no right or wrong way to react to news of a loved one's death. One never really knows what the relationship has been like and no assumptions should be made. Facts need to be given without suggesting a response. "It's a blessing. He could never have led a normal life after this," may be a helpful rationalization coming from the family, but is inappropriate from caregivers. Likewise, "Now don't overreact; be strong" is less helpful than "You will get through this and there will be people to help." The health professional is not expected to do something to alleviate the family's pain at this time, but only to stay with family members as they experience the gamut of emotions.

3. Let the family ask questions. In the immediate shock of receiving news of the death of a loved one, some questions may seem inappropriate. They may reflect denial or total disbelief, anger, or inability or unwillingness to comprehend. No questions are inappropriate.

4. Answer questions simply and with honesty. This is not the time for complicated medical facts or hypotheses about what has happened. All known information does not have to be given at this time, and information may have to be repeated. Whether the patient was conscious and/or likely to have been in pain are common pressing issues for the family.

5. After family members have had time to collect themselves, and as soon as possible, offer them the opportunity to be with the deceased. Most experts agree that viewing the body exerts a beneficial influence on the acutely grieving family—creating a reality of death (3). Persons who cannot tolerate seeing the patient will usually say so. While some regret viewing the body of a loved one, more regret *not* having seen the loved one in the ER (3). Rarely will the medical team have to make the decision not to allow viewing given the nature of the injuries.

Family members need to be prepared for the viewing by receiving information about what they will see and by being given time to prepare themselves before the viewing. Some want the presence of clergy; others may need to call other family members to be with them for the viewing. In all cases, it is useful for a member of the hospital team to view the body just before the family does, and thus to be able to accurately describe to them exactly what they will see. Turning down the glaring lights of the ER and setting an appropriate scene can do much to create an atmosphere of warmth. Extraneous machinery can be removed from the room and chairs should be available in case a family member feels faint or wants to sit quietly for a period.

The ER staff must realize that the family will relive for months the words and actions of the staff and review for a lifetime the events of that day. There is no need to hurry this moment.

6. While viewing the body, some may want to be silent and others can be helped by being directed to talk about the person who has died. Prayers may be appropriate or some families may benefit by being asked to share aloud a memory of the deceased. While it may seem strange to a beginning practitioner, families have routinely reported that it is helpful to be asked about the deceased person. It may be perceived as caring to ask a grieving son or daughter: "I didn't get to know your mother, can you tell me about her?" Asking a few details about his wife might facilitate a distraught husband to engage and focus for a few minutes. While tears often come with the storytelling, the recollections can bring unity to those present and are a comforting part of the work of grieving.

7. After family members have had a chance to view the body, they may require very specific instructions about how to proceed. The fact that they will have to go home alone has often not yet occurred to them. Step-by-step talking through of the necessary next actions is helpful. Discuss how they will get home, who will be there, who should be called, when to call to make funeral arrangements, and how they will get through the next hours.

8. Family members can be given the names and numbers of local crisis teams or other places where emergency psychological support may be available in case they are needed. The normalcy of grief reactions should be briefly discussed. An ER phone number and the name of a staff member whom they can call with any forgotten questions is useful. The family may need to wait at the hospital for other loved ones to arrive or for others to come and provide support before they can go home.

9. After the family leaves, it is helpful to designate one member of the ER team to call the family later to see how it is coping and to answer any remaining questions. Many families will then want to review details, ask if their loved ones had said any last words, or ask again if they had suffered from their injuries before dying.

10. When there has been a death in the ER, the team of caregivers also needs an opportunity to review the events and to share feelings associated with the trauma and with coping with the family. (See the chapter, "Psychological Support and Care of the Staff.")

Telling Patients About the Death of Others in the Accident

ER staff and family members often agonize over when and how to tell an injured person of the death of others in the same traumatic event. The patient may be asking about the others. While we can appreciate the reluctance on the part of all concerned to "burden" an injured person with bad news, the patient often has a strong suspicion about reality. To give false information to patients or avoid the questions may only escalate their worry. We feel that the sooner the patient is told the reality, the sooner others can rally to support the patient. The following case examples illustrate some typical reactions of the patient to the death of others at the scene.

CASE STUDY 1

A mother, an 18-month-old infant, and a grandmother were in a house fire where mother and grandmother were burned trying to save the child who died. Family members tried to protect the grandmother from the knowledge of the child's death. They were afraid the trauma would kill her. The next day the grandmother learned of the death from a newspaper article in the paper. When the family finally talked honestly with the grandmother, she said, "I knew little Jennifer could not be alive or I would have heard her cry because the burns really hurt. When no one talked about her I thought it was because you blamed me for her death and were going to punish me by never talking about her again." Such misunderstandings can be avoided when the truth is told.

CASE STUDY 2

A 54-year-old man and his 28-year-old daughter were hit by a car while riding bicycles. The man was unconscious when brought to the ER but soon awoke and asked about his daughter, who had been killed. The doctor advised that the family not tell him and in fact told the patient that his daughter was injured but would be fine. The family went along with the pretense but felt increasing anxiety as they were forced to keep up a cheerful demeanor in front of the patient. A day after the funeral for the daughter, the father was told about the death of his daughter by his wife and son. While they had not wanted to "burden" him with the news, he was furious at their betrayal and deeply resented that he had not been given the opportunity to grieve with the rest of the family and to participate in the funeral plans.

There may be times when a patient's medical condition is so unstable that doctors do not want a death discussed. As soon as the patient is stabilized, however, the issue should be raised. When the patient does ask, we support truthful answers.

What to Tell Children About Death

The question of how to tell children about death often comes up in the ER. While it is perfectly natural for adults to take a protective attitude toward children, children are acutely sensitive to changes in emotional climate and, in general, tend to be aware of change before they understand the particulars of what has happened. In the absence of explanations about what is really going on in the adult world, a child is likely to make up his own explanations of what is happening. Children are usually capable of dealing with loss in ways that surprise adults.

CASE STUDY 3

An 11-year-old boy and his mother were in a car accident. The car had burst into flames and the mother died trapped in the car; the son managed to escape through a window but sustained burns over 30% of his body. When the father visited the ER and learned of his wife's death, he insisted his son not be told about his mother and he, in fact, lied to the child, saying that she had some burns but was okay. After a few hours, the injured boy became increasingly agitated and uncooperative with his care and started screaming to see his mother. The father was helped to see that the child needed a truthful explanation, and he told the child of the death of his mother. "I knew she couldn't have lived because she was still in that car. When I thought of her alive and burned, I was very frightened." Father and son were able to begin their grief and the child was calm and cooperative.

The life of the family is built around emotional experiences, good and bad. When good things happen they are shared and when sad things happen they also need to be shared. Even the most uncomfortable feelings can be faced openly. To be lied to while he is faced with an emotional climate that he cannot fully understand is a double injury to a child.

Parents tend to know their child best and their instincts regarding what to tell their child can usually be supported. Some suggestions may be helpful. In general, the idea of going to sleep forever should be avoided with children. It can lead to fears about not waking up. Parents can be asked what prior experiences the child has had with loss and then be advised to build on that knowledge.

The age of the child being told about death will affect how the child is told and what reaction one can expect. Children's definitions of what death means differ according to their age. Preschoolers often think that death is a reversible process, like falling asleep and waking up or going away for a time and returning. After the age of 6 years, children are usually better able to understand the finality of death, but may not fully comprehend the fact that it will eventually happen to everyone, including themselves. Between the ages of 6 and 9 years, children sometimes think that death is contagious and may avoid someone they think or have heard is dying. Youngsters between 9 and 12 years understand what happens when a person dies but may worry more about what they said or did to cause this to happen. Pre-adolescents and teens may get caught up in the practical arrangements and issues related to death (4).

Children usually do not focus on the loss for as long a time as adults do, and parents need to be warned that their child may seem initially to be unaffected and to want to return to play. It is in their play over the many months ahead that they will work through their grief reactions.

It is not wrong for children to see the emotions of adults around them, although they may need reassurance about the reason for tears or protection from constant exposure to the display of feelings. The problem is how to be honest with our own feelings and, at the same time, to be able to provide the child with a sense of security. Adults can help a child recognize the difference between sadness and despair, and understand that reasonable expression of feeling is different from complete collapse. The child can be spared the extreme evidence of adult breakdown but should be given explanations such as, "I am sad because your grandmother has died and won't be with us any more." This is quite different from, "Stop asking questions and run along. It is nothing that concerns you and you are too young to understand."

For children of all ages it is normal to have a sense of guilt about the death of a loved one. They need to be told directly that death cannot be caused by negative thoughts about a person.

Some hospitals have a brochure they give to parents about dealing with death at various ages. Religious groups may have resources to offer families, and funeral homes often have pamphlets about the psychological needs of children in the midst of a traumatic event or death. Schools have resources for the school-aged child. It is important to make clear to families immediately that children need to be included in the grieving process and that there is help available for them. As in the case of adults, children need permission to grieve at their own time and in their own fashion.

References

1. Titchener JL. Management and study of psychological response to trauma. J Trauma 1970;10:974–980.
2. Imbus SH, Zawacki B. Autonomy for burned patients when survival is unprecedented. N Engl J Med 297:308–311, 1977.
3. Parrish GA, Holdren KS, Skiendzielewski JJ. Emergency department experience with sudden death: a survey of survivors. Ann Emerg Med 1987;16:1792–796.
4. Jackson EN. Telling a child about death. New York: Hawthorn/Dutton, 1965.

3

Organic Mental Syndrome

When working with patients in a mental, general, or specialized hospital, one must constantly be alert to the presence of organic mental syndrome (OMS). Nowhere is this truer than with injured patients who may not only have direct damage to the central nervous system (CNS), but may also be candidates for OMS due to underlying medical disease, metabolic disturbances, medications, and the effects of intensive care on the sensory system. The proper diagnosis of OMS is essential; it leads to a search for the underlying etiology and insures a timely treatment when the cause is reversible. Proper diagnosis also allows the staff to prepare for variations in patient behavior that might be harmful to the patient. For example, the patient might fall and be hurt or try to climb out of bed and add to his or her injuries. A patient with OMS might not be able to cooperate for blood drawing, radiography, debridement, or casting, and may try to pull out IV lines or an endotracheal tube. When the presence of OMS is recognized and the etiology is known, the staff and family can be prepared for the expected clinical course.

OMS is frequently misdiagnosed in the medical setting. Bizarre and confused behavior is written off as an emotional reaction. This is especially true if the patient has a psychiatric history or if the patient is believed to be eccentric in any way. We have found that medical students are able to learn the basic difference between "psychotic" and "confused." But somehow, when students progress to housestaff and beyond, the differential is forgotten. Hopefully, this chapter will clarify these issues.

Classifications and Conceptual Framework

In the current diagnostic nomenclature (DSM III-R), OMS refers to a constellation of psychological or behavioral signs and symptoms without reference to etiology. These symptoms are listed under the Classification of Organic Mental Disorders Associated with Axis III Physical Conditions or

Conditions Whose Disorder Is Unknown (Table 3.1). While the criteria listed under the definitions for delirium (Table 3.2) are used by many, the criteria are definitive and fairly strict. These requirements could be a limiting factor in the critical care setting, where the staff need to understand that there may be an OMS even if full criteria for delirium are not met.

Table 3.1. DSM III-R Classification of Organic Mental Disorders Associated with Axis III Physical Conditions or Conditions Whose Disorder Is Unknown[a]

Code	Classification
293.00	Delirium
294.10	Dementia
294.00	Amnestic Disorder
293.82	Organic Hallucinations
293.83	Organic Mood Disorder (specify: manic, depressed, or mixed)
294.80	Organic Anxiety Disorder
310.10	Organic Personality Disorder
294.80	Organic Mental Disorder (not otherwise specified)

[a] Reprinted with permission from the *Diagnostic and Statistical Manual of Mental Disorders.* 3rd ed., Revised. Copyright 1987, American Psychiatric Association.

Table 3.2. Diagnostic Criteria for Delirium[a]

A. Reduced ability to maintain attention to external stimuli (e.g., questions must be repeated because attention wanders) and to appropriately shift attention to new external stimuli (e.g., perseverates answer to a previous question).
B. Disorganized thinking, as indicated by rambling, irrelevant, or incoherent speech.
C. At least two of the following:
   (1) reduced level of consciousness, e.g., difficulty keeping awake during examination
   (2) perceptual disturbances: misinterpretations, illusions, or hallucinations
   (3) disturbance of sleep-wake cycle with insomnia or daytime sleepiness
   (4) increased or decreased psychomotor activity
   (5) disorientation to time, place, or person
   (6) memory impairment, e.g., inability to learn new material, such as the names of several unrelated objects after 5 min, or to remember past events, such as history of current episodes of illness
D. Clinical features develop over a short period of time, (usually hours to days) and tend to fluctuate over the course of a day.
E. Either (1) or (2):
   (1) evidence from the history, physical examination, or laboratory tests of a specific organic factor (or factors) judged to be etiologically related to the disturbance
   (2) In the absence of such evidence, an etiological organic factor can be presumed if the disturbance cannot be accounted for by any nonorganic mental disorder, e.g., Manic Episode accounting for agitation and sleep disturbance.

[a] Reprinted with permission from the *Diagnostic and Statistical Manual of Mental Disorders.* 3rd ed., Revised. Copyright 1987, American Psychiatric Association.

Table 3.3. Diagnostic Criteria for Dementia[a]

A. Demonstrable evidence of impairment in short- and long-term memory. Impairment in short-term memory (inability to learn new information) may be indicated by inability to remember three objects after five minutes. Long-term memory impairment (inability to remember information that was known in the past) may be indicated by inability to remember past personal information (e.g., what happened yesterday, birthplace, occupation) or facts of common knowledge (e.g., past Presidents, well-known dates).
B. At least one of the following:
 (1) impairment in abstract thinking, as indicated by inability to find similarities and differences between related words, difficulty in defining words and concepts, and similar tasks
 (2) impaired judgment, as indicated by inability to make reasonable plans to deal with interpersonal, family, and job-related problems and issues
 (3) other disturbances of higher cortical function, such as aphasia (disorder or language), apraxia (inability to carry out motor activities despite intact comprehension and motor function), agnosia (failure to recognize or identify objects despite intact sensory function), and "constructional difficulty" (e.g., inability to copy three-dimensional figures, assemble blocks, or arrange sticks in specific designs)
 (4) personality change, i.e., alteration or accentuation of premorbid traits
C. The disturbance in A and B significantly interferes with work or usual social activities or relationships with others.
D. Not occurring exclusively during the course of Delirium.
E. Either (1) or (2):
 (1) there is evidence from the history, physical examination, or laboratory tests of a specific organic factor (or factors) judged to be etiologically related to the disturbance
 (2) In the absence of such evidence, an etiologic organic factor can be presumed if the disturbance cannot be accounted for by any nonorganic mental disorder, e.g., Major Depression accounting for cognitive impairment

[a] Reprinted with permission from the *Diagnostic and Statistical Manual of Mental Disorders.* 3rd ed., Revised. Copyright 1987, American Psychiatric Association.

Table 3.4. Criteria for Severity of Dementia[a]

Mild: Although work or social activities are significantly impaired, the capacity for independent living remains, with adequate personal hygiene and relatively intact judgment.

Moderate: Independent living is hazardous, and some degree of supervision is necessary.

Severe: Activities of daily living are so impaired that continual supervision is required, e.g., unable to maintain minimal personal hygiene; largely incoherent or mute.

[a] Reprinted with permission from the *Diagnostic and Statistical Manual of Mental Disorders.* 3rd ed., Revised. Copyright 1987, American Psychiatric Association.

Technically, the criteria for dementia (Tables 3.3 and 3.4) are not met if the symptoms only occur with a reduced ability to maintain or shift attention to external stimuli, as in delirium. Delirium and dementia can co-exist. The criteria for dementia are of special value in evaluating patients in the rehabilitation phase of treatment.

The DSM III-R official code is presented because of its prime importance in creating a data base for intraprofessional communication. The specific criteria for each category are defined in DSM III-R. However, in the clinical setting, and especially with acute burn and trauma patients, we prefer that the more general term, *organic mental syndrome*, be utilized. The reason is that a single etiology for OMS can rarely be determined. Also, a simple presentation is unlikely. It is important to be aware of the wide range of changing symptoms as well as of the varying etiologies that occur in this setting.

It is recognized clinically that brain functions are lost in the order opposite to that in which they are acquired, both in the life history of the individual and in the development of the species. Higher functions are lost before lower functions, which are thus released from higher control. This approach recognizes the work of John Hughlings Jackson (1), who conceptualized a hierarchically arranged CNS. With loss of function at one level, function on the next level emerges unrestrained by the integrating and inhibitory influence of the higher centers.

Jackson reported that organic brain disorders produce both negative and positive symptoms. The negative ones are due to the loss of function, while positive ones develop as other structures or functions compensate for the loss. Anatomically, it seems that negative signs are produced by the depression of cortical functions, while positive signs are due to the release of limbic structures from cortical inhibition (2). Table 3.5 delineates the negative

Table 3.5.   Negative Signs of Organic Mental Syndrome[a]

CNS Function Impaired	Sign of Impairment
Cognition	Ability to abstract, retention and recall, recent memory, orientation, and remote memory are all affected
Level of consciousness	Concentration span affected, apathy, lethargy, somnolence, stupor, coma
Motor functions	Ataxia, slurred speech, asterixis, tremor, myoclonic twitching, incontinence

[a] Modified from Glickman LS. Psychiatric consultation in the general hospital. New York: Marcel Dekker, Inc., 1980:57.

losses of OMS, and Table 3.6 shows the positive signs, with impairment of ego function due to cortical damage and subsequent release of emotions controlled by lower senses of the brain. This clinical picture will also be influenced by the psychological response to injury, which is a part of the personality and not necessarily a function of a damaged brain, but rather a psychological response to a damaged brain (see chapter 4, "Psychological Reactions").

CLINICAL DIAGNOSIS OF ORGANIC MENTAL SYNDROME

The patient with OMS will usually appear sufficiently confused or show easily recognizable memory deficit, suggesting the appropriate diagnosis. As previously noted, it is important not to misinterpret such a response as a manifestation of emotional difficulties. In cases where the clinical picture is subtle or is perhaps at an early stage, diagnosis is more difficult. Familiarity with the clinical course, as well as with a wide variety of diagnostic tests and techniques, is helpful. The diagnostic criteria for delirium and dementia have been stated in Tables 3.2 and 3.3, and the clinician should be alert for signs or symptoms that suggest OMS. We describe the early and later, full-blown, manifestations below.

It is important that the clinical findings that make the diagnosis of OMS be documented in the medical record. This is particularly necessary because the condition is dynamic. There is value in comparing changes in the mental state over time or as other variables, such as medications, are changed.

Early Organic Mental Syndrome

Minimal anxiety, apprehension, and restless agitation may be the earliest manifestations of OMS. Intermittent and slight disorientation may or may not be detected. Patients know who they are and where they are, but may not know the day or time. Disorientation usually progresses from difficulties with sense of time and day to uncertainty about place. Disorientation to

Table 3.6.   Causes of Positive Signs of Organic Mental Syndrome[a]

Ego Functions Impaired	Positive Signs Produced
Repression	Anxiety, agitation
Suppression, social judgment, impulse control	Socially unacceptable sexual and aggressive behavior
Reality testing	Hallucinations, delusions

[a] Modified from Glickman LS. Psychiatric consultation in the general hospital. New York: Marcel Dekker, Inc., 1980:58.

person is rare, and occurs in advanced OMS. The patient may have intermittent periods of lucidity during this time. Abnormalities in sleep patterns can occur early and be intermittent. There may be either difficulty in falling asleep or early morning awakenings. Patients may report agitation about dreams and nightmares. They may not be sure whether they were asleep or awake when they had these dreams, confusing them with reality. The patient may have difficulty understanding the full meaning of a conversation and may show evidence of trying to cover up this deficit. Repeated questions asked by the patient about his or her illness, or about anything else, may suggest these memory gaps. Ability to assimilate information or learn simple tasks may point to cognitive inabilities that can appear in OMS even while orientation is clear (3).

If a patient becomes agitated and anxious when asked to do a cognitive or simple memory task, this is almost always diagnostic of OMS. This agitation appears to be a defensive reaction to the realization of the deficit. It is probably the progenitor of catastrophic reaction (4), which is pathognomonic for OMS. In situations with alcohol withdrawal, one of the earliest manifestations may be the presence of an auditory click that the patient reports hearing. Or patients report that they see a shimmering screen in front of their eyes. The patient's general physical condition may be deteriorating at this point and may be reflected in physical and laboratory findings.

Frank Organic Mental Syndrome

At this time, there would usually be a clear disorientation for time and place. The patient is obviously confused. Agitation may be quite severe. Visual hallucinations may occur; these are rare in nonorganic functional psychosis. Visual hallucinations in a non-OMS patient usually involve a religious delusion. Auditory hallucinations are about half as common as visual hallucinations in patients with OMS (5). Tactile hallucinations are rare, but when they occur in patients with OMS, they are more likely related to an alcohol problem. Olfactory hallucinations are the rarest, but are known to occur with certain brain lesions. The patient with frank OMS often pulls on his or her hospital gown, and misinterprets cues in the immediate surroundings. The patient believes, for example, that his bed sheets are clothes or that a table is a machine. Patients concoct gross confabulations to make up for significant memory gaps. A patient may say he has seen you before, or that he was at home during the night. There can be paranoid delusions which, as the OMS progresses, become less organized and easily forgotten.

NEUROPSYCHOLOGICAL TESTING

Numerous formal and informal tests can document OMS. These tests give numerical results that can be compared during various points in the hospital course. The scores may demonstrate improvement or other variations helpful to the medical and surgical team and, at times, may be meaningful to the patient and family. The Folstein Mini-Mental State (Appendices A and B) and the Jacobs Cognitive Capacity Screening Examination (Appendix C) are examples of such tests.

A variation of these tests that we have used in the burn unit is the Burn Unit Delirium Scale (BUDS) (Table 3.7). It can be adapted for the trauma unit as the Trauma Unit Delirium Scale (TUDS). At the beginning of our liaison activity in the burn unit, we encouraged the nurses to obtain a BUDS score on every patient, on a regular basis. We would regularly ask them the latest BUDS score. With the cooperation of the burn unit surgeons, we incorporated these scores into the regular rounds. For a period of time, the entire staff would discuss the BUDS score (along with the vital signs, electrolytes, blood gas numbers): "The BUDS score was 28, up 4 points from the previous day." Or, "The evening BUDS score was elevated to 32 from 16 during the day." These data would flow together with other important data, and were easily accepted into the everyday functioning of the unit. Sometimes this would include the Visual Analog Pain Scale score for pain evaluation (see chapter 1, "Pain").

We have found that, despite the value of the scores and their easy acceptance, it is not necessary to run these tests on a regular basis. The staff learns to pick up the signs and symptoms of OMS, and the effort expended for formal testing on a regular basis is not always an efficient use of time. On units where a psychiatric team makes rounds on a regular basis, the entire unit can be attuned to making the diagnosis of OMS. Time spent in documentation might better be directed to psychological care of the patient.

Another useful and easy screening test to document OMS on the record is the Draw-a-Clock Test (6-8). Our method is, first, to ask the patient to name a wrist watch as we point to this object ("What is this?"). The question not only tests the ability to understand verbal commands and screens for aphasia, but also orients the patient to the task at hand. The patient is then handed a paper showing a circle, approximately 3–5 inches in diameter, with a dot in the middle. The patient is given a pencil and asked to draw a clock with all the numbers and the hands of the clock pointing out a specific time, such as 10 after 3.

Table 3.7. Burn Unit Delirium Scale (BUDS)

PATIENT NAME: _____ DATE: _____ SHIFT: _____
NURSE: _____

INSTRUCTIONS: Check the items which are answered incorrectly. If any of the items change during the course of the shift (i.e., pt. becomes confused) you may correct the score.

SUGGESTED INTRODUCTION FOR THE INITIAL TESTING: "I would like to ask you a few questions. Some you will find easy and others may be very hard. Just do your best."

I. *Orientation to time, place and person:*
   1. "What is the month?"   1. _____
   2. "What is the date?" (correct if ±5 days)   2. _____
   3. "What is the year?"   3. _____
   4. "Where are you?"   4. _____
   5. (Check if you observe that the patient is unable to recognize
      familiar people i.e. primary nurse, family)   5. _____

II. *Calculations:*
   6. (Choose four random numbers e.g. 8-1-4-3)
      "Listen to these four numbers 8-1-4-3. Count 1 to 10 out loud and
      then repeat 8-1-4-3."   6. _____
   7. "Repeat the numbers which you have just said backwards?"   7. _____
   8. "9 + 3 is"   8. _____
   9. "Add 6 to your answer."   9. _____
  10. "Take away 5"   10. _____

      (Each time you give this question to the patient you may choose
      other comparable numbers to minimize learning effect.)

III. *Perceptual Illusions:*
  11. "Some people who have burn injuries see or hear things and
      wonder if they are real. Have you seen or heard things in the past
      24 hours which seemed strange or unusual to you?"   11. _____

IV. *Dreams:*
  12. "Did you have any unusually vivid dreams last night?"   12. _____

V. *Hallucinations:*
  13. "During the past 24 hours have objects, voices, sounds, colors or
      smells appeared out of nowhere or have you seen or heard things
      which are not there?"   13. _____

VI. *Paranoid Ideation:*
  14. "During the past twenty four hours have you had the feeling that
      people are making you suffer on purpose or that people are talking
      about you behind your back?"   14. _____

                                        Add the total of items checked:
                                                  Total # wrong: ‾‾14‾‾

During the testing the patient was: (Check as many as apply. Do not count in the above score)
Cooperative _____ Uncooperative _____ Depressed _____
Lethargic _____ Other-Specify _____

[a] Blumenfield M, Reddish P. Burn unit. Westchester County Medical Center, 1982.

Most patients, even including those with significant degrees of OMS, attempt this task with surprisingly little anxiety or resistance. As long as they are physically capable of attempting the motor task (can use their hands) and understand the command, most patients will not appear threatened by this request. We do not use a formal scoring system, but find it easy to group patients' drawings into categories of mild, moderate, or severe

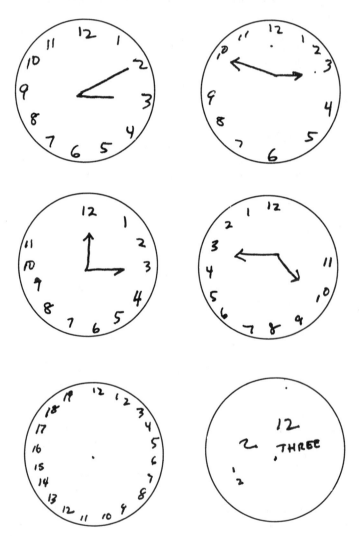

Figure 3.1.   Examples of responses to a clock drawing test: "Draw a clock with the time ten after three."

impairment (Fig. 3.1). Patients may forget the time told to them, demonstrating a short-term memory deficit in addition to the spatial motor deficits illustrating OMS. Comparison at a later date can demonstrate dramatic improvements in patients with a reversible OMS etiology, or deterioration in other cases. By asking patients to sign their names, the ability to write is also observed. Variations in handwriting will also show up as the patient improves or worsens. We also find this a good graphic demonstration to place in the chart, and often include this test along with our written consultations.

Formal neuropsychological testing can be performed by a psychologist trained in this area and may be useful in the later phase of the hospitalization when there is permanent brain damage or head injury. This can be helpful in localizing brain damage and documenting functional disability. Among these tests are the Halsted-Reitan Neuropsychological Test Battery, which can give a fairly good assessment of the level of brain dysfunction. It can require up to 2 full days to administer these tests and can be difficult to use in the general hospital. The Luria-Nebraska Neuropsychological Battery consists of 14 scales that provide information on motor, tactile, and intellectual functioning as well as an assessment of receptive and expressive language abilities. Localization scores and factor scores allow more exact identification of deficit areas. This test requires 2–4 hours to administer (9).

Search for the Specific Etiology of OMS

Once OMS is diagnosed or even suspected by the psychiatrist and psychosocial team, it is important that the other members of the medical team be directed toward confirming this diagnosis and, wherever possible, determining the exact etiology of it. The concomitant presence of disorders such as psychosis, depression, anxiety, anger, personality disorders, and so forth should not delay or deter any effort to make the proper diagnosis of OMS and, especially, to rule out any reversible etiology. It sometimes can happen that inexperienced medical staff become less likely to pursue the underlying diagnosis of OMS when psychiatric diagnosis or psychological symptoms are apparent. In such a situation, it must be pointed out that it is highly unlikely that OMS would be caused by purely psychological reactions.

Obviously, a careful history and physical examination, including a detailed neurological examination, are essential in working up an OMS. The determination of any localizing signs that point to a central brain injury will suggest that the OMS and localizing symptoms are being caused by a lesion usually related to the trauma. It is possible, however, that the localizing signs and symptoms are caused by a lesion and that the OMS may be caused by still another organic factor.

A complete battery of laboratory tests should make it possible to rule out any metabolic factors, including electrolyte and thyroid abnormalities, liver and renal impairments, and B-12 or folic acid deficiency. Some deviations from normal, such as sodium and potassium levels, can be rapidly corrected and ruled out as the underlying causes of OMS. In the critical care setting, blood gases can be closely monitored, and it should be easily understood that poor gas exchange is an etiological factor for OMS.

It is well known that the presence of infection, with particularly high fever and sepsis, causes delirium and OMS. When there is a brain abscess or meningitis, OMS is, of course, often a presentation. Treatment with antibiotics and the subsequent improvement of fever and decrease in the white count will usually correlate with the improvement of OMS in this situation.

The patient history should give suggestions of prescribed medications that may have caused changes in mental status. Drug interactions should always be considered. As discussed in Chapter 1, "Pain," as well as in Chapter 6, "The Use of Psychotropic Drugs," pain medications can act synergistically with psychotropic drugs such as benzodiazepines and others that have a tendency to sedate. Therefore, there can be a resulting typical picture of confusion. Morphine and meperidine (Demerol), as well as other drugs given for pain can also cause a classic OMS. Sometimes this occurs with one class of medications in a particular patient and will not occur with another group of pain medications. Changing medications may sometimes alleviate the problem.

The presence of drugs, including alcohol, in toxic doses or that interact with various other medications can cause OMS. Drug or alcohol withdrawal syndrome can also cause OMS. This is discussed in Chapter 7, "Alcohol and Substance Abuse." It is important to note that a drug toxicology and alcohol blood and urine screen is always useful in detecting substances that may be causing an early picture of OMS.

Steroids given to minimize edema of the brain or taken for certain medical conditions or by athletes or body builders can cause OMS as well as other psychiatric symptoms.

It has been consistently observed by us and others that patients with significant burns (more than 25% total body surface area) will often develop OMS with a characteristic delirium. This will usually begin at day 7 to 10 and will often last up to 2 weeks or more (or until the burns are all healed or grafted) before going into remission. We have seen this occur despite the fact that no organic factor has been determined. Such a delirium is not correlated with a dosage level or even with the presence of a particular medication for pain.

There are two other situations, common in the intensive care setting, that can produce a clinical picture resembling or even identical to OMS, but that are not yet related to a direct and clear organic etiology. The first situation is sleep deprivation, which has been demonstrated to cause abnormal brain wave patterns and thus may have some indirect organic basis. The other common intensive care setting situation that can resemble OMS are either sensory deprivation or sensory overload. The isolation of the patient from the awareness of night and day, the covering eyes and prevention of visual stimuli, the steady beeping sound of equipment—which prevents other auditory input—and the prevention of movement by traction and other apparatus are all examples of sensory deprivation. Overload occurs when there is a never-ending activity around the patient with numerous people, procedures, information, and so forth. Both situations have been shown to lead to a clinical picture identical to OMS. Some of the new intensive care beds, which constantly move portions of the mattress to prevent pressure sores, have a steady electronic and mechanical sound that can be particularly bothersome to the patient and can lead to manifestations of OMS as well as other psychiatric symptoms. Similarly, a revolving or swinging bed frame that constantly moves the patient can lead to these clinical manifestations.

In the 1990s, no discussion of the etiology of OMS is complete without mention of the possibility of AIDS. Patients who are HIV positive can show evidence of OMS. The history of being in a high risk group or of having other evidence of the disease will suggest this diagnosis. This will be discussed later in Chapter 9, "The Impact of AIDS."

HEAD OR BRAIN IMAGING

When available, computerized axial tomography (CAT) and magnetic resonance imaging (MRI) allow visualization of the brain and detection of traumatic injuries that were never previously visualized. In CAT scanning of the brain, thousands of low-dose x-ray readings are computer processed to yield cross-sectional images. Consecutive cross-sections can be used to generate a three-dimensional image of the brain. In the MRI, a magnetic field is applied to the brain. The aligning and relaxation of exposed hydrogen atoms (protons) as influenced by pulses of radio frequencies produce energy that is used to construct images of the brain. This technique allows brain structures to be clearly visualized (10).

CAT scans better visualize bone and high-density material and the MRI is better suited for soft tissue visualization, but either can be quite helpful. Both procedures require some cooperation on the part of the patient. MRI requires more cooperation from the patient, and patients who are highly anxious or confused may not tolerate being placed in the narrow chamber necessary for the procedure. MRI procedures remain quite costly due to the specialized equipment.

CASE STUDY 1

A 30-year-old man with a head injury sustained in a motor vehicle accident showed mild episodes of confusion with decreased attention span. He became agitated when his cognitive ability was tested. The CAT scan at the level of the frontal and temporal lobe showed bilateral hemorrhages (white, high attenuation areas) in the frontal lobes and diffuse cerebral edema (dark, lower attenuation areas) in both the frontal and temporal lobes (Fig. 3.2).

CASE STUDY 2

A 56-year-old woman who suffered multiple fractures and head injury was hospitalized for several months. She was initially in a coma and then showed gradual improvement of mental status with a residual OMS. An MRI study at the level of the vertex showed areas of gliosis that have increased signal (arrowheads) and hemosiderin deposition (arrows), which are seen as areas of low signal intensity (Fig. 3.3).

ELECTROENCEPHALOGRAM

The electroencephalogram (EEG) measures the brain's electrical activities through electrodes placed in standard positions on the scalp. The largest contribution to the EEG recording originates from the neurons in the cortex. An abnormal EEG may distinguish organic from functional brain disorders. Deviation from the normal EEG pattern usually indicates underlying brain pathology. For example, an abnormally slow wave activity in the awake state could reflect a specific structural abnormality if localized or could reflect a diffuse dysfunction if generalized (10). Comparing serial EEGs can demonstrate a gradual return to normal activity, which could reflect a healing process even before it shows up in the clinical picture.

Serial EEGs may also be of prognostic value regarding the prospect of epilepsy. Sharp waves or spikes sometimes emerge as the focal slow wave

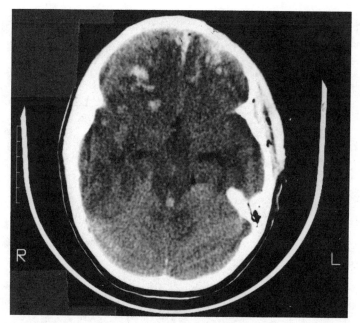

Figure 3.2. CAT scan at the level of the frontal and temporal lobes of a man who had a head injury in a motor cycle accident, and who showed mild episodes of confusion with decreased attention span. Not the bilateral hemorrhages (white, high attenuation areas) in the frontal lobes and diffuse cerebral edema (dark, lower attenuation areas) in both the frontal and temporal lobes. CAT scan study courtesy of Michael Tanner, M.D., Professor and Chairman, Department of Radiology, New York Medical College, Valhalla, NY.

abnormality resolves and may precede the occurrence of posttraumatic epilepsy (11).

OTHER TESTS

Lumbar puncture (LP) and the examination of the cerebral spinal fluid are not currently used as first-line tests in the work-up of a trauma patient with OMS because of the availability of the newer, previouosly described brain imaging techniques, which are less invasive. If the cerebral spinal fluid pressure is high, as evidenced by headache and papilledema, an LP may pose a risk to the patient. When it is appropriate to perform an LP, information can be obtained to assist the diagnosis of subarrachnoid hemorrhage, meningitis, and other neurologic diseases (10).

There are many other traditional diagnostic tests that may be used by neurologists in working up the differential diagnosis of OMS. These include

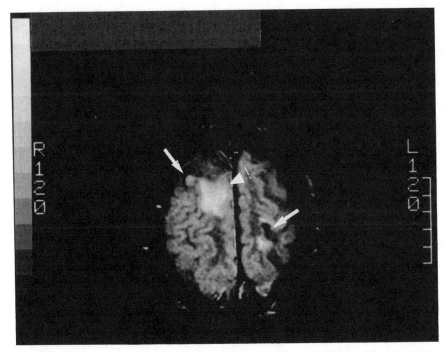

Figure 3.3. An MRI study at the level of the vertex of a woman who suffered multiple fractures and head injury. She was in a coma and then showed gradual improvement of mental status with a residual OMS. Note the areas of gliosis that have increased signal (arrowheads) and homosiderin deposition (arrows), which are seen as areas of low signal intensity. MRI Study courtesy of Michael Tanner, M.D., Professor and Chairman, Department of Radiology, New York Medical College, Valhalla, NY.

angiography, pneumoencephalography, ventriculography, myelography, ultrasound. CAT and MRI have often made these tests unnecessary.

Newer procedures such as computerized evoked potentials, brain imaging by positron emission tomography (PET), and single photon emission computed tomography (SPECT), as well as neuroendocrine and other biochemical tests, may also be used on a more regular basis in the future.

Management of the Patient with OMS

As soon as the early signs of OMS are noted, and even before an investigation into possible etiologies begins, management interventions should be initiated with the patient.

AGITATION

The first priority in any patient presenting with OMS must be safety (12). When confusion, agitation, and inappropriate behavior prevail, the patient requires protection from falls, wandering, pulling out I.V. tubing or other necessary equipment, and possibly hurting others. Use of side rails on the bed and soft restraints are adequate controls for some patients; others benefit from being placed on constant awareness or frequent awareness status.

While mild, unagitated confusion may be easily tolerated in a patient, more pronounced confusion and agitation will require a low-dose neuroleptic or antipsychotic, such as haloperidol (Haldol), administered orally or parentally. A dose of 2–10 mg may be needed to obtain an initial response, and then 0.5–2.0 mg b.i.d. may be adequate (13). In rare situations, larger doses combined with benzodiazepines, such as lorazepam, along with close monitoring may be necessary. Because evening symptoms of OMS are often more pronounced, 1–5 mg Haldol at bedtime may be necessary. Neuroleptics should not be used on a p.r.n. basis but should be ordered at regular intervals and tapered and stopped as soon as symptoms of OMS clear (14). This type of medication is, of course, appropriate when there are psychotic manifestations such as hallucinations, paranoid ideation, or other delusional thoughts. For more information, see also Chapter 6, "The Use of Psychotropic Drugs."

DISORIENTATION

Increased confusion and disorientation toward evening should be anticipated, and the room should be arranged and lighted, if possible, to avoid shadows and total darkness. Behavior must be more closely observed at night and reassurances about environmental stimuli may need to be more frequent. While a normalized sleep and wake cycle is important, CNS depressants should be avoided as sleep aids; they tend to further aggravate the mental state of the patient. Use of relaxation, back rubs, warm milk, and, if needed, a low dose of phenothiazine to aid sleep is preferable (15, 16). Bedtime rituals that are consistent and include personal care—freshening up of the bed for sleep, nightclothes from home if appropriate—and any of the patient's normal bedtime routines, as learned from the patient or family, can help.

Disorientation to sequence and time can be helped through the use of easily seen wall clocks and up-to-date calendars in each room. The nurse and other caregivers can provide clear verbal indications about the time of day, seasonally appropriate activities, and events that are going on in the world.

To minimize disorientation to place, the patient should be moved as little as possible from room to room and belongings from home should be utilized where practical. With each interaction patients can be reminded where they are and what is going on around them. Patients who are repeatedly asked the name of the hospital may become agitated with this task and might better be matter-of-factly told where they are in casual conversation until their mentation has clearly improved.

While patients with OMS usually know who they are, limiting the number of professionals caring for them can decrease their confusion as to person. The nurse can facilitate the patient's recall by stating his or her name and by stating in simple terms what is going to be done. The patient needs to be told what is expected of him or her. Asking the patient to make even simple choices may not be appropriate at this time and might only increase patient frustration. Pictures of loved ones placed in the room and frequent, regular (even if short) visits by a few family members or close friends or family can help reorient the delirious patient. It may be useful to always address the patient by his or her most familiar name without infantilization. While a 27-year-old "Jonathan" may be accustomed to be called "John" by his friends and "Johnny" by his parents, it would be a mistake for caregivers to utilize the diminutive form that might evoke regression in the patient (14).

SENSORY OVERLOAD OR DEPRIVATION

To help the OMS patient make sense of the environment, one must first optimize the patient's use of the senses by making certain glasses, hearing aids, false teeth, and other assistive devices are available and in working condition. Caregivers need to be seen and heard by the patient and need to document the patient's needs to assure shift-to-shift consistency. In some cases, the room may be rearranged so that people will enter on the side closest to the patient's "good ear" or closest to the eye with better vision.

Sensory overload is most acute when there is constant lighting, over-crowding with invasion of personal space, and unpleasant or loud noise (17). Each patient varies in noise tolerance. Noises that create expectation of something unpleasant or untoward, such as the sound of the dressing cart in the burn center or the x-ray machine being rolled through the ICU, can be particularly upsetting and cause the patient unnecessary anxiety if the treatments expected are not for them. Control over noise factors is important and patients should be asked if they want the radio or television on or off and whether the volume is adjusted to their satisfaction. Sometimes a patient will not even realize the toll of a particular noise until it is removed. Noisy beds and alarms or machines that make continuous noise should be turned off at intervals when possible. A patient reported to like country music may not want it played continuously, and a favorite tape is not a favorite for long if played on every shift.

Understimulation becomes a problem for the delirious patient who is on a ventilator or is phasing in and out of consciousness. Caregivers frequently forget to talk to the patient. Even if it is uncertain that the patient can hear and interpret what is said, and independent of whether the patient can respond, all patients should be talked to (18). Persons giving care should identify themselves and explain in simple terms what they are going to do.

As soon as it is medically feasible, the removal of a burn or trauma patient from the ICU surrounding can bring the most dramatic recovery from OMS (13). A change of scene, the presence of a window that records the change from light to dark, the sense of getting well again, and a more normal environmental setting with a less pressured and stressful atmosphere, can produce what seems like a miracle in the recovery from delirium.

PERSONALITY CHANGES

Patients with OMS are not themselves; there are factors that control their thoughts, feelings, and behaviors. It is vital that all persons caring for such a patient keep this point in mind and abstain from impatience, punishment, or avoidance as a way of handling undesirable behavior. It is easy to become annoyed with tangential, irrelevant, boisterous conversation, and repetitive and often dangerous behavior. The patient with OMS, however, needs to be free of negative labels and needs to be approached with every ounce of creativity and positive energy to get through this difficult period or to adjust to any permanent damage.

OMS DUE TO ALCOHOL AND DRUGS

Alcoholic patients who present with symptoms of obtundation in the early phase of treatment may receive 100 mg thiamine i.m. to prevent or reverse a deficiency encephalopathy (19). They, of course, also need a detoxification protocol as will patients who have been abusing certain drugs. This is discussed in Chapter 7, "Alcohol and Substance Abuse."

Traumatic Head and Brain Injury

Head trauma statistics have skyrocketed since the development of high-speed automobiles. Transport-related events produce by far the largest number of head traumas with resultant brain injury every year. Falls and assaults are the distant second and third leading causes of head trauma (20). Peak incidence for this injury is between the ages of 15 and 24, with large numbers also concentrated in infants and children and in the elderly.

The brain can be injured by blunt or nonpenetrating injuries just as it can be injured by penetrating injuries. While it is difficult to predict the long-term prognosis for recovery based on the level of consciousness or clinical presentation during the initial hospitalization, several trends have been noted to have value in predicting specific outcomes. A poor outcome is seen in patients who during initial hospitalization have impaired bilateral pupillary response, physical underactivity, and prolonged agitation, or who are elderly. Also, the duration of posttraumatic amnesia is correlated with subsequent cognitive recovery (21).

While, in 1974, the Glasgow Coma Scale was talked about widely as a predictor of outcome in head trauma (22), later studies have emphasized psychosocial factors. An overly pessimistic attitude on the part of the caregivers and family may negatively affect outcome, while an overly optimistic outlook may not affect the outcome (23). Although coma scales are still widely used, outcomes remain difficult to predict with certainty. Severity of injury, preinjury behavior and personality of the injured, and psychosocial adversity—including family and living setting—affect outcome (24).

PERSONALITY CHANGES

In addition to cognitive deficits already described in this chapter, the head injured person often has an intensification of preexisting personality traits such as disorderliness, suspiciousness, argumentativeness, isolationism, disruptiveness, and anxiety (21). Some of these behaviors may be due to a cortical dysinhibition or cortical release phenomena; the injured part of the brain can no longer control the emotional responses that originate in the lower centers of the brain. Because of the vulnerability of the prefrontal and frontal regions of the cortex to injury, specific changes in personality, known as the frontal lobe syndrome, are not uncommon in head and brain injuries. These changes include decreased motivation, impaired social judgment, and labile affect. Patients may display uncharacteristic lewdness, inability to appreciate the effects of their behavior or remarks on others, a loss of social graces, a lack of attention to personal appearance, and boisterousness. In addition, impaired judgment may be prominent and may take the form of dimished concern for the future, an increase in risk-taking behavior, and unrestrained consumption of alcohol. Such patients may appear shallow, indifferent, or apathetic, with a global lack of concern for the consequences of their behavior. This syndrome is labeled organic personality in DSM III-R (25).

In instances of organic personality disorder, the cognitive function of the patient may be preserved, leading to the impression that the patient is showing only a psychological reaction to the injury. Abnormal findings on tests such as EEG, brain imaging, and others will suggest that the personality changes are at least in part due to an organic etiology.

It has been suggested that the two hemispheres of the brain appear to contribute differently to the psychological sequelae after traumatic brain injury (26). The right hemisphere is specialized both to perceive and to express emotion, so that emotional stimuli are comprehended more accurately when they are able to gain access to this hemisphere of the brain (27). Adult patients after right-hemisphere brain injury, therefore, have difficulty understanding the emotional tone of what people say. They also have difficulty communicating emotion and, in general, appear apathetic or indifferent to emotions and even euphoric (24). Patients with left hemisphere brain lesions tend to appear depressed and anxious. They are usually able to express their emotion (28).

Most of the time the full significance of alterations in personality will not be apparent until after the acute medical and surgical condition has stabilized. This may be weeks, months, or even a year or more after the patient has been discharged from the acute care hospital.

Personality changes due to brain and head injury are often also part of a syndrome with several names such as posttraumatic nervous instability, postconcussive syndrome, and others (29). Headache, which can have onset at any time in the posttrauma period and is of a variable nature, is the central symptom. It is either generalized or localized to a part of the head which was struck. Dizziness may be another prominent symptom. The patient is often intolerant of noise and emotional excitement. This syndrome may be mistaken for anxiety and depression, which are reactions to the trauma. Indeed, with time, there will be an intermixing of organic mental changes and purely psychological responses, and the two can often not be clearly delineated.

In children who sustain head and brain trauma, the personality changes are not so clear due to the fact that personalities are forming and developing. Parents are likely to report that their child does not act like himself or is displaying a "bad disposition" (30).

MAJOR PSYCHIATRIC DISORDERS

Just as there can be an intensification of preexisting personality traits occurring secondary to head injury, there can also be an exacerbation of preexisting affective illness of both depressive and manic types. Affective illness not previously known to be present can develop. There may be an exacerbation of an underlying schizophrenia.

Recent studies have demonstrated that either left anterior cortical or subcortical lesions may lead to the development of major depression and that preexisting subcortical atrophy may play an important permissive role in the development of major depression. On the other hand, mania has been associated with damage to the right hemisphere. Preexisting subcortical atrophy and genetic vulnerability may also play important roles (31).

The development of psychotic symptoms as part of OMS has been discussed earlier. There is the possibility that such symptoms may be associated with posttraumatic seizures that develop in 5% of patients with closed head injuries and in 50% of those with compound skull fractures (29). Ninety-nine percent of such seizures occur 1 to 3 months after injury, and therefore will not show up during the acute hospitalization period of most patients. Mention of the possibility of seizures may be helpful in preventing panic in some families, but would only add to the anxiety of others.

AGGRESSION

In a review of 26 patients with severe traumatic closed head injury, 25 exhibited more than one episode of agitated behavior in the acute period after the trauma (32). Explosive and violent behavior can be an important clinical manifestation of focal brain lesions as well as of diffuse damage to the central nervous system. Such behavior may be beyond the aggression that is part of the personality changes or any underlying psychiatric disorder.

Silver and colleagues have described an organic aggressive syndrome (21). They found that the standard use of antipsychotic drugs and benzodiazepines, described in the chapter on psychotropic medication, may not always be sufficient. They reviewed the literature that suggested the use of anticonvulsants such as carbamazepine for the treatment of organic aggressive syndrome, and also discussed the use of β-adrenergic blocking agents such as propranolol for the treatment of uncontrolled rage and violent outbursts secondary to brain damage. The doses to which patients responded were generally lower than 640 mg/day, with a median dosage of 100 mg/day. Responsiveness varied from less than 2 days to more than 6 weeks for therapeutic effect. They also cautioned about combining drugs with thioridazine (Mellaril), which could be raised to toxic levels in combination.

Corrigan and Mysiw point to the period of pronounced confusion and agitation in the head trauma patient as representing a discrete state of recovery from the traumatic injury. They point out that cognitive function may improve before agitation. Thus, drugs designed to control aggression and agitation may decrease cognitive function and, therefore, prolong agitation (33).

In one study of head-injured adults, 70% continued to have difficulty with anger control 5 years after injury, with little or no abatement over time. One can imagine the adjustments this would require for patient and family (34).

IMPACT OF HEAD INJURY ON FAMILY

The adjustments to be made by the patient and family following head injury deserve special mention. While the course and recovery of intellectual functioning over the first 6–12 months is often impressive, with a more gradual improvement in later stages, subtle changes in memory and attention may continue for up 2 years and impose major constraints on quality of life. Memory deficits, reduced speed of information processing, and inflexibility in problem solving are all problems to overcome and will be quite apparent during the initial hospitalization. Levin reports, however, that "of the range of neurobehavioral sequelae, psychiatric manifestations produce the greatest burden and stress in families" (35).

In other studies, research has shown that emotional disability secondary to head injury is more difficult for families to deal with than physical disabilities (36). The greatest concern of relatives when there is a head injury appears to be about predicting the course of personality changes (37). That estimate cannot be made during the early phase of hospitalization. Thus, there is an enormous element of uncertainty for the head-injured patient and family.

In addition to adjusting to emotional disturbances in their loved ones, there are often shifting roles due to disability. Spouses lose their emotional support and companionship and are faced with isolation and loneliness. Return to work may be impaired due to intolerance of employers or real physical and emotional disabilities. Mild verbal problems may be no problem for the mechanic, but may pose major obstacles for the patient who is a lawyer. Disinhibition may mean unemployment for the diplomat while it may not be recognized in a homeless person (38).

Persons recovering from head trauma may be considered unmotivated or uncooperative when, in fact, because of injury to frontal lobes, they have lost the ability to initiate purposeful activity. Damage to the limbic system deep inside the brain distorts emotions and physical desires; impulsive sexual behaviors can result in exhibitionism and hypersexual episodes. Aggression resulting from temporal lobe damage is typically unprovoked and abrupt. Damage here may cause poor memory and difficulty in new learning, thus affecting a person's ability to relearn appropriate behaviors (39). With the addition of any of these changes to a family member, the entire family can rapidly be in crises.

In a separate chapter, we discuss support of the family of burn or trauma patients.

References

1. Jackson H. Selected writings of John Hughlings Jackson. New York: Basic Books Inc., 1958.
2. Glickman LS. Psychiatric consultation in the general hospital. New York: Marcel Dekker, Inc., 1980.
3. Sullivan N, Fogel BS. Could this be delirium? Am J Nurs 1986;1359–1363.
4. Goldstein K. The effect of brain damage on the personality. Psychiatry 1952;15:245–260.
5. Schwab JL. Handbook of psychiatric consultation. New York: Appleton-Century-Crofts, 1968.
6. Critchley M. The parietal lobes. New York: Hafner Press, 1953;172–202.
7. Wolf-Klein GP, Brod MSA, Silverstone FA, et al. A rapid screening test for Alzheimer's disease. Gerontologist 1987;27:21.
8. Wolf-Klein GP, Silverstone FA, Fevy AP, Brod MS. Screening for Alzheimer's disease by clock drawing. J Am Geriatr Soc 1989;37:730–734.
9. Franzen M, Lovell MR. Neuropsychological assessment. In: Hales RE, Yudofsky SC, eds. Textbook of neuropsychiatry. Washington: American Psychiatric Press, 1987:41–55.
10. Rosse RB, Owen CM, Morihisa JM. Brain imaging and laboratory testing in neuropsychiatry. In: Hales RE, Yudofsky SC, eds. Textbook of neuropsychiatry. Washington: American Psychiatric Press, 1987:17–40.
11. Adams RD, Victor M. Special techniques for neurologic diagnosis. In: Principles of neurology. 3rd ed. New York: McGraw Hill, 1985:10–35.
12. Baggerly J. Rehabilitation of the adult with head trauma. Nurs Clin North Am 1986;21:577–586.
13. Kleck H. ICU syndrome; onset, manifestations, treatment, stressors, and prevention. Crit Care Q 1984;21–28.
14. Trockman G. Caring for the confused or delirious patient. Am J Nurs 1978;78:1495–1499.
15. Beck C. Mental health—psychiatric nursing: a holistic life cycle approach. St. Louis: CV Mosby, 1984.
16. Davidhizar R, Gunden E, Wehlage D. Recognizing and caring for the delirious patient. J Psychiatr Nurs Ment Health Services 1978;38–41.
17. Baker CF. Sensory overload and noise in the ICU: sources of environmental stress. Crit Care Q 1984;66–79.
18. LaPuma J, Schiedermayer D, Gulyas A, et al. Talking to comatose patients. Neurotrauma Medical Report 1990;4:1–3.
19. Blankfein R. Delirium. Hosp Physician 1984;23–32.
20. Cooper PR, ed. Head Injury. 2nd ed. Baltimore: Williams & Wilkins, 1987.
21. Silver JM, Yudofsky SC, Hales RE. Neuropsychiatric aspects of traumatic brain injury. In: Hales RE, Yudofsky SC, eds. Textbook of neuropsychiatry. Washington: American Psychiatric Press, 1987;179–190.
22. Teasdale G, Jennett B. Assessment of coma and impaired consciousness: a practical scale. Lancet 1974;2:81–84.

23. Gianotta S, Weiner J, Karnaze D. Prognosis and outcome in severe head injury. In: Cooper PR, ed. Head injury. 2nd ed. Baltimore: Williams & Wilkins, 1987:464–489.
24. Lehr E. Psychosocial issues. In: Lehr E, ed. Psychological management of traumatic brain injuries in children and adolescents. Rockville, MD: Aspen, 1990:155–185.
25. American Psychiatric Association. Diagnostic and statistical manual of mental disorders. 3rd ed, revised. Washington: American Psychiatric Association, 1987.
26. Bryden MP, Ley RG. Right hemispheric involvement in the perception and expression of emotion in normal humans. In: Heilman KM, Satz P, eds. Neuropsychology of human emotions. New York: Guilford Press, 1983.
27. Gianotti G. Laterality of affect: the emotional behavior of right and left brain damaged patients. In: Gianotti G, ed. Hemisyndromes: psychobiology, neurology, psychiatry. San Diego: Academic Press, 1983.
28. Goldstein K. The effect of brain damage on the personality. Psychiatry 1952;15:245–260.
29. Adams RD, Victor M. Craniocerebral trauma. In: Adams RD, Victor M, eds. Principles of neurology. 3rd ed. New York: McGraw Hill, 1985.
30. Prigatano G. Neuropsychological rehabilitation after brain injury. Baltimore: Johns Hopkins University Press, 1985.
31. Robinson RG, Starkstein SE. Mood disorders following stroke: new findings and future directions. J. Geriatr Psychiatry 1989;22:1–15.
32. Rao N, Jellinek HM, Woolston DC. Agitation in closed head injury; haloperidol effect and rehabilitation outcome. Arch Phys Med Rehabil 1985;66:30–34.
33. Corrigan JD, Mysiw J. Agitation following traumatic head injury: equivocal evidence for a discrete stage of cognitive recovery. Arch Phys Med Rehabil 1988;69:487–492.
34. Lezak MD. Relationships between personality disorders, social disturbances, and physical disability following traumatic brain injury. J Head Trauma 1987;2:57–69.
35. Levin H. Neurobehavioral sequelae of head injury. In: Cooper PR, ed. Head injury. 2nd ed. Baltimore: Williams & Wilkins, 1987:442–463.
36. Pauting A, Merry PA. The long-term rehabilitation of severe head injuries with particular reference to the need for social and medical support for the patient's family. Rehabilitation 1972;38:33–37.
37. Oddy M, Humphrey M, Uhley D. Stress upon the relatives of head injury patients. Br J Psychiatry 1978;133:507–513.
38. Vinkes P, Bruyn G, Klawans H, eds. Handbook of clinical neurology—Head injury. Amsterdam: Elsevier, 1990.
39. Out of control—the behavioral effects of head injury. Headlines—The Brain Injury Magazine. [From New Medico Head Injury System] Compiled from interviews with Sperling K, Burke W, Hagen C, Russo D, Isenberg N. Spring, 1990.

APPENDIX A. The Folstein Mini-Mental State Examination[a]

Patient _____

Examiner _____

Date _____

Maximum Score	Score	
		Orientation
5	( )	What is the (year) (season) (date) (day) (month)?
5	( )	Where are we (state) (county) (city) (hospital) (floor)?
		Registration
3	( )	Name 3 objects (1 second to say each). Then ask pt. all 3 after you have said them. Give 1 point for each correct answer. Then repeat them until pt. learns all 3. Count trials and record. Trials _____
		Attention and Calculation
5	( )	Serial 7's. 1 point for each correct. Stop after 5 answers. Alternatively, spell "world" backward.
		Recall
3	( )	Ask for the 3 objects repeated above. Give 1 point for each correct.
		Language
9	( )	Name a pencil, and name a watch. (2 points) Repeat the following: "No ifs, ands, or buts." (1 point) Follow a 3-stage command: Take a paper in your right hand, fold it in half, and put it on the floor." (3 points) Read and obey the following: Close your eyes. (1 point) Write a sentence. (1 point) Copy design. (1 point)
30	( )	Total score

Assess level of consciousness along a continuum:

Alert	Drowsy	Stupor	Coma

[a] Adapted with permission from J Psychiatr Res 12, Folstein MF, Folstein SE, McHugh PR. "Mini-mental state," a practical method for grading the cognitive state of patients for the clinician. Copyright 1975, Pergamon Press PLC.

APPENDIX B. Instructions for Administration of the Mini-Mental State Examination[a]

Orientation

- Ask for the date. Then ask specifically for parts omitted, e.g., "Can you also tell me what season it is?" One point for each correct.
- Ask in turn "Can you tell me the name of this hospital?" (city, county, etc.). One point for each correct.

Registration

- Ask the patient if you may test his/her memory. Then say the names of 3 unrelated objects, clearly and slowly, about 1 second for each. After you have said all 3, ask pt. to repeat them. This first repetition determines score (0–3) but keep saying them until all 3 can be repeated, up to 6 trials. If pt. does not eventually learn all 3, recall cannot be meaningfully tested.

Attention and Calculation

- Ask the pt. to begin with 100 and count backward by 7. Stop after 5 subtractions (93, 86, 79, 65). Score the total number of correct answers. If the pt. cannot or will not perform this task, ask pt. to spell the word "world" backward. The score is the number of letters in correct order, e.g., "dlrow" = 5, "dlorw" = 3.

Recall

- Ask the pt. to recall the 3 words previously asked above to test memory. Score 0–3.

Language

- Naming: Show the pt. a wrist watch and ask what it is; repeat for pencil. Score 0–2.
- Repetition: Ask the pt. to repeat the sentence after you. Allow only one trial. Score 0 or 1.
- 3-stage command: Give pt. a piece of plain blank paper and repeat the command. Score 1 point for each part correctly executed.
- Reading: On a blank piece of paper print the sentence "Close your eyes" in letters large enough for the pt. to see clearly. Ask pt. to read it and do what it says. Score 1 point only if pt. actually closes his eyes.
- Writing: Give the pt. a blank piece of paper and ask pt. to write a sentence for you. Do not dictate a sentence; it is to be written spontaneously. It must contain a subject and a verb and be sensible. Correct grammar and punctuation are not necessary.
- Copying: On a clean piece of paper, draw intersecting pentagons (each side about 1 in.) and ask pt. to copy it exactly. All 10 angles must be present, and 2 must intersect to score 1 point. Tremor and rotation are ignored. Estimate the pt's. level of sensorium along a continuum, from alert on the left to coma on the right.

[a] Adapted with permission from J Psychiatr Res 12, Folstein MF, Folstein SE, McHugh, PR. "Mini-mental state," a practical method for grading the cognitive state of patients for the clinician. Copyright 1975, Pergamon Press PLC.

APPENDIX C. Jacobs Cognitive Capacity Screening Examination[a]

Examiner _____ Date _____

Instructions: Check items answered correctly. Write incorrect or unusual answers in space provided. If necessary, urge pt. once to complete task.

Introduction to pt.: "I would like to ask you a few questions. Some you will find very easy and others may be very difficult. Just do your best."

1. What day of the week is this? _____
2. What month? _____
3. What day of month? _____
4. What year? _____
5. What place is this? _____
6. Repeat the numbers 8 7 2. _____
7. Say them backward. _____
8. Repeat the numbers 6 3 7 1. _____
9. Listen to these numbers 6 9 4. Count 1 to 10 out loud, then repeat 6 9 4. (Help, if needed. Then use numbers 5 7 3.) _____
10. Listen to these numbers 8 1 4 3. Count 1–10 out loud. Then repeat 8 1 4 3. _____
11. Beginning with Sunday, say the days of the week backward. _____
12. 9 + 3 is _____
13. Add 6 (to previous answer or "to 12"). _____
14. Take away 5 ("from 18"). Repeat these words after me and remember them. I will ask for them later: HAT CAR TREE TWENTY-SIX _____

15. The opposite of fast is slow. The opposite of up is _____
16. The opposite of large is _____
17. The opposite of hard is _____
18. An orange and a banana are both fruits. Red and blue are both _____
19. A penny and dime are both _____
20. What were those words I asked you to remember? (HAT)
21. (CAR)
22. (TREE)
23. (TWENTY-SIX)
24. Take away 7 from 100, then take away 7 from what is left and keep going: 100 − 7 is _____
25. Minus 7 _____
26. Minus 7 (write down answers; check correct subtraction of 7) _____
27. Minus 7 _____
28. Minus 7 _____
29. Minus 7 _____
30. Minus 7 _____

TOTAL CORRECT (maximum score = 30)

Patient's occupation (previous, if not employed): _____

Education _____ Age _____

Estimated intelligence (based on education, occupation, and history, not test score): Below average, Average, Above average.

Patient was: Cooperative _____ Uncooperative _____ Depressed _____ Lethargic _____ Other _____

Medical Diagnosis: _____

If pt.'s score is less than 20, the existence of diminished cognitive capacity is present. Therefore, an organic mental syndrome should be suspected and the following information obtained:

Temp. _____ BUN _____ Endocrine dysfunction? _____

B.P. _____ Glu _____ T_3, T_4, Ca, P, etc.

Hct _____ PO_2 _____ History of previous psychiatric difficulty _____

Na _____ PCO_2 _____ Drugs: _____

K _____ Steroids? *L*-Dopa? Amphetamines? Tranquilizers?

Cl _____ Digitalis?

CO_2 _____ Focal neurological signs: _____

EEG _____ _____

ECG _____ DIAGNOSIS: _____

_____

a Modified, with permission, from Jacobs JW, Bernhard MR, Delgado A, Strain JJ. Screening for organic mental syndromes in the medically ill. Ann Intern Med 1977;86:40.

4

Psychological Reactions

A trauma or burn injury is almost always an unexpected event. The brave fire fighter does not expect to be seriously injured and cannot be psychologically prepared for trauma. Even the person who has inflicted a self-injury in a suicide attempt does not anticipate the aftermath of the injury. Only the rare person who has had a previous severe injury or multiple trauma will immediately understand the physical and emotional travail that will have to be faced.

With significant injury comes significant pain. The response of the patient and staff to the pain and the effects of the medication given for pain relief all have a major impact on the patient's psychological response. Chapter 1 in this book emphasizes the primary position that we have assigned to understanding and treating pain in the trauma and burn patient.

The impact of the injury on the central nervous system also influences the psychological response of the patient. The presence of a clouded sensorium, disinhibited cortical function, and of *cognitive deficits* all affect the psychological experience of the injured patient. As previously described, medication, anesthesia, sensory deprivation and overload, as well as sleep deprivation all affect the ultimate psychological response.

Conservation Withdrawal

During the acute phase of severe injury there is often an initial period of withdrawal. This withdrawal is more likely to occur with a large burn, loss of limb, or serious threat to life, although the reaction is common to the majority of injured patients. Children, in particular, are likely to exhibit this behavior (1).

The withdrawing patient shows little interest in external events, family, or friends. The patient's affect is blunted and may even be judged inappropriate, especially in the presence of a major loss or injury. This is probably due to a combination of physiological conservation-withdrawal reaction and an ego defense mechanism of denial.

A conservation-withdrawal response is a psychophysiological state characterized by decreased interaction with the environment, decreased energy, decreased activation of bodily systems, and immobilization (2, 3). Frequently, there is a decrease in heart rate, blood pressure, and even body temperature, as well as diminished muscle tone and a decrease in the general level of motor activity. This is caused by an activation of the parasympathetic system. There may be other physiological events that mask these autonomic changes in the physically injured patient.

Conservation withdrawal often subsides within 1 or 2 weeks after the injury, but may persist when there is a sustained physiological threat to the patient's life. The preoccupation with pain, dressing changes, traction, blood drawings, and ventilators appears to take up most of the physical and psychological energy of the patient. During the early stages of an injury, this withdrawal response is often mistaken for depression. However, at this point, the patient rarely communicates ideation compatible with depression. The patient's thoughts have not yet integrated the "big picture," which comprises the consequences that the injury will have on his or her life. There may be little interest in others nearby who are injured. The patient often sleeps whenever possible, keeping his or her eyes closed most of the time and mainly responding to issues of pain and comfort. Usually, in the early phase of an injury, this response will not interfere with resuscitation after burn injury or the initial acute phase of trauma care. There is little reason to force communication at this point. Family members may be distressed when they see this significant withdrawal response. However, if the patient is progressing well medically, the family can be assured that the emotional state will soon change with the improvement of the physical condition.

In a severe injury that requires continuous critical care, withdrawal may persist for weeks or, rarely, even with good physical recovery, for months. In such cases, the distinction between withdrawal conservation and depression may be difficult to make. When there is sustained withdrawal, more vigorous treatment with psychostimulants, antidepressants, or psychological intervention should be considered. Treatment of depression will be discussed in a later chapter.

Denial

In the early phase of injury, if communication with the patient is possible, it may become apparent that the patient is utilizing the defense mechanism of denial. This is more likely to occur in patients who have had disfigurement or loss of limb, but is also part of the psychological response repertoire of most trauma and burn patients as well as of all those who have a serious physical illness. A patient can deny the extent of an injury, the loss of a body part, the loss of function, the loss of life or injury to others, or the loss of home or other significant property. The patient may acknowledge the loss of limb, but will not show the expected concern about this major loss. The patient may not ask about loved ones who were in the accident. Or, if he knows the facts, may not have an obvious grief response. A patient with significant disability, who talks about expectations to go home or return to work in a short time, is most likely utilizing the defense mechanism of denial.

Denial is a protective, unconscious defense mechanism. It relieves anxiety that arises when an individual is threatened with the possibility of death, mutilation, and pain. The reduction of anxiety has a protective value for the psychological self or ego, as does conservation withdrawal. Similarly, reduced anxiety causes a reduction of catecholamine response, which may protect the heart (3).

A physical analogy of denial occurs in the pupillary response to light (4). To avoid overstimulation of the retina by too much light, the iris contracts. In the same way, the defense mechanism of denial protects the person from too much psychological stimulation caused by a frightening perception of an external reality.

The surgical team frequently sees denial as a pathological process based on unreality. The surgeons may attempt to remove the denial by a forced confrontation in reality testing, or may ask the psychological team to "fix" the problem by removing the denial. The abrupt removal of denial in the early phase of an injury may disrupt a vulnerable ego, leading to marked anxiety, a narcissistic rage, severe depression, and even overt psychosis. With time, most often one to two weeks after pain is controlled, denial usually gives way to reasonable reality testing. However, it may take many months or years before a severely injured person fully understands and accepts new limitations.

Allowing a patient to maintain denial during the early stages of care following injury does not mean giving him false hope or misinformation about his condition. Patients who use denial do not usually ask questions and, frequently, do not hear information given to them. Patients should always be encouraged to ask questions and should be given information in doses over time or as requested. However, this does not mean forcing upon them a reality for which they are unprepared.

Denial becomes dangerous for the patient when it prevents him or her from making an important reality assessment that is necessary for safety or realistic future planning. A person utilizing denial may want to sign out of the hospital, refuse essential medication or a necessary surgical procedure, or try to make an important decision. When this happens, the patient using denial may be confronted by staff who have an ongoing, positive relationship with him or her and who will be in a position to do some firm reality testing. When possible, an important family member should be part of this discussion. Frequent follow-up is necessary after such a discussion so that the patient can react and ask questions. Although follow-up visits may be quite brief, it would be a mistake to confront the patient with an issue that he or she is denying and then neglect to follow up on that issue on the same or the next day. A sedative or tranquilizer is not a substitute for a follow-up visit after such a confrontation.

If psychiatrists or other mental health professionals are available, it is understandable that the surgical team may ask them to handle the patient's denial. It is more desirable, however, that this defense mechanism be confronted jointly by the surgical, nursing, and mental health team.

Regression

Most patients who are hospitalized and seriously injured demonstrate some degree of psychological regression: They return to an earlier way of coping with stress. The patient often must be completely cared for by the medical and nursing staff. This facilitates a regressed psychological state. Patients can be assertive, demanding, and have temper tantrums. They may be tearful and cling to a dependence relationship even when capable of doing things for themselves. The developmental anxieties mentioned below help to precipitate a regression to an earlier childhood pattern of adaptation, as does forced passivity and the dependence that the patient develops toward his or her caretakers (4). At the same time as the patient engages in regressive behavior, he can have guilt feelings about that behavior.

As described above, in the section on denial, there is no value in verbally attacking the patient for regressive behavior. It should be recognized that the staff sometimes views regressive behavior as provocative and manipulative. Staff members can easily be angered by this kind of behavior. They may be tempted to utilize some form of behavior modification with negative rewards: leaving the patient in a soiled sheet in order to teach him or her a lesson, or purposely delaying their response to a call. Such responses are inappropriate because the regressed state is initially experienced by the patient as a reality. It is more effective for the staff to recognize that the patient feels like a child. The patient needs the support and the extra care *and* the encouragement to become gradually more independent. Further discussion of the treatment of regression is covered in the chapters on treatment and on family involvement.

Anger and Hostility

At any point along the way from injury to full recovery, anger and hostility may be experienced by the trauma and burn patient. The successful recognition and handling of anger is an integral part of the care of any such patient.

Averill states that, on the psychological level, anger is aimed at the correction of some appraised wrong (5). Perhaps the most obvious basis for anger is loss or threatened loss and the resulting grief response. The patient has temporarily lost control and may have also lost limbs, body image, possessions, loved ones. Minimally, the sense of invulnerability that most people carry around is at least temporarily lost and familiar surroundings as well as loved ones are absent. Clothes have been taken away. Control over urination has probably been removed, at least initially, due to the need to catheterize the patient in order to monitor output. Even the act of breathing on one's own may have been lost.

Patients show angry, agitated feelings for a variety of reasons. The differential diagnosis of this behavior should always be addressed. Acute pain that requires attention and correction of undermedication should be a prime consideration in the angry and agitated patient. Organic mental syndrome with subsequent confusion and agitation should be recognized and corrected when possible. Head injuries can cause changes in behavior patterns, with anger and agitation constituting an important part of the presenting picture. Substance abuse may present with agitation, anger, and hostile feelings on the part of the patient. Withdrawal syndrome, particularly from alcohol and drugs—which are topics discussed later in this book—needs to be recognized and treated. The side effects of medication can also be a factor in the presentation of anger and agitation. An adjustment of dosage or a change to a different drug may be indicated.

Patients who have a persistent, major psychiatric disorder may, as part of their usual behavior pattern or during a psychotic decompensation, show agitated, angry, and even paranoid behavior. In such situations, psychotropic medication is usually appropriate.

It is probable that angry and agitated behavior is universal in persons who are hospitalized with trauma or burn injury. These individuals have experienced loss or threatened loss, and anger is part of the grief response.

In the case of the burn and trauma patient, anger is usually first seen in the emergency room and, later, as the patient assumes the dependent role of the injured. The patient may or may not be aware of angry feelings and may repress them, turn them inward as depression, or express them. The next chapter discusses the delicate approach for dealing with displaced anger that has been redirected from the self to the medical staff and the family. The anger may be expressed at the actual target of anger or, more commonly, projected or displaced onto another person.

Anxiety

Another common emotion of burn or trauma patients is anxiety. To better understand the patient, it is useful to view this feeling from a developmental and psychodynamic perspective.

Anxiety emerges because the person experiences the injury as a dangerous situation that reawakens basic fears and threats encountered during early childhood development. These fears have been delineated by Strain and Grossman (6, 7). While there may be some conscious awareness of feelings of anxiety, feelings of anxiety come, for the most part, from the unconscious. The anxiety may be related to a trauma and burn injury in the ways described below.

BASIC THREAT TO NARCISSISTIC INTEGRITY

Injury and hospitalization challenge the universal, irrational, and narcissistic belief that a person must always be capable, independent, and self-sufficient. After a burn or trauma injury, the patient no longer perceives himself as being fully intact. The sense of wholeness is violated. The infantile fantasy persisting in adulthood—the fantasy of the omnipotent parent or the doctor or nurse ensuring a pain-free, pleasurable protected existence and immortality for the patient—has been seriously questioned.

FEAR OF STRANGERS

In the hospital, the patient must put his or her life in the hands of strangers. They put the patient to sleep, operate on him or her, and care for all bodily needs. They are aliens whose actions arouse very early insecurities concerning "stranger anxiety." These insecurities have their origin in human development between the third and sixth months of life, when the infant becomes fearful of a stranger's face.

FEAR OF SEPARATION

Hospitalization leads to separation from family and friends. This brings out "separation anxiety," which has its origin in the child's early separation from his or her mother, normally occurring between the ages of 6 and 30 months. The anxiety is reenacted several times subsequently as the child begins to attend school and, ultimately, years later, lives alone. There will be great variation in the ability of patients to tolerate separation from loved ones. Since a hospitalization for traumatic injury can be long, some patients become quite anxious about the extended separation.

Being seriously injured also brings out fears about death and dying. To most, death means a separation from loved ones, thus the emotions mobilized by thoughts about death are a form of separation anxiety.

FEAR OF LOSS OF LOVE AND APPROVAL

Patients who are injured and burned are greatly concerned about losing their attractiveness and ability to perform their usual activities. This fear may lead to concerns that they will lose the love, respect, and approval of family, friends, and peers. The origin of this anxiety goes back to the age of about 2 years, when the child realizes that all his needs may not be automatically gratified by his or her mother. Subsequently, the developing child realizes that fulfillment of needs is contingent, in part, on the ability to please parents and others.

FEAR OF LOSS OF BODY PARTS OR OF INJURY TO THEM

Any injury to any area of the body can reawaken concern regarding the loss of body integrity and, in particular, it can reawaken derivatives of "castration anxiety" in males and "mutilation anxiety" in females. These fears are derived from childhood, when the 2- to 3-year-old child discovers the anatomical difference between the sexes. This leads the young child to anxiously contemplate that a loss of genitals has occurred or might occur. Injuries or surgery, especially during childhood, can make a person especially sensitive to this type of anxiety. Patients hospitalized with a trauma or burn injury have their bodies exposed, probed, and weakened, making them quite susceptible to a reawakening of this anxiety. The anxiety can occur with any injury, but may be more enhanced with injuries to the eyes, face, genitals, and breasts.

FEAR OF LOSS OF DEVELOPMENTALLY ACHIEVED FUNCTION

Injury can cause a loss of control of bowel, bladder, or motor and sensory function, either on a temporary or permanent basis. This real or anticipated loss leads to great anxiety relating to the regressed state. There can be an exaggerated concern that a transient loss will become permanent. Of course, some patients will have to face this reality.

FEAR OF RETALIATION

As described below, the injury may be experienced as a punishment for previous transgressions—some sins of omission or commission. These emotions may bring forth feelings of guilt and shame that were felt during earlier stages of life.

Such anxiety and fear may also be related to the regressed state, described above. When, as a small child, the child regressed and lost previously gained sphincter control, there might have been some reprimand or punishment from parents. In a similar manner, the injured patient may fear retaliation from physicians and nurses.

Depression

A depressed mood or depressed feelings are expected responses to any loss or threatened loss. Injury may involve loss of body function and of family and work roles. All of the fears noted above that bring anxiety also involve some degree of loss and, therefore, can also bring about depressed feelings. Depression manifests itself in many ways. Patients may verbalize sadness; they may weep overtly or have a sad facial expression. Decreased appetite, weight loss, sleep disturbances, and, particularly, early morning awakenings and diminished psychomotor activity are hallmarks of a depressed mood.

Because a physically traumatic injury, particularly a burn injury, brings about many metabolic changes, it is often difficult to diagnose a depressed state solely from vegetative signs and symptoms.

The distinction between *grief* and uncomplicated bereavement, which may include a depressed mood and *depression*—which is a part of a more serious depressive syndrome or disorder—is often hazy. The distinction may, however, be important in deciding which supportive and therapeutic approach to utilize with the patient (8). In the usual presentation, the grieving patient does not have a significant decrease in self-esteem. The patient realizes that the injury has caused temporary or permanent losses and limitations; the patient does not feel less lovable as a person and has not lost the belief that he or she deserves the affection and attention of others. The grieving person feels sad and depressed and is in a depressed mood.

We begin to consider that the injured person has progressed to a depressed condition when the loss caused by the trauma or burn becomes distorted in the person's mind and when there is a concomitant decrease in the patient's sense of worthiness as a person. Instead of a preoccupation with memories, sadness about loss, and rumination about real issues, the more seriously depressed patient begins to give the loss a meaning that damages self-esteem. The amputee views himself as "just a cripple" or the burned patient views herself as "a disfigured nobody." These feelings can be accompanied by irrational guilt, harshly punitive self-accusations, and feelings of helplessness and hopelessness that are magnified beyond the restrictions posed by the injury. The presence of significant vegetative symptoms, such as sleep disturbances, constipation, diminished appetite, decreased sexual desire, and a generalized slowing are more likely with significant depression. However, these symptoms do occur in the grieving patient, and are likely secondary manifestations of the patient's physical condition when there is a major injury.

The specific criteria in DSM III-R should be consulted when the presence of an actual mood disorder is suspected.

It is always wise to look for a history of previous mental illness, especially a major affective disorder, since depression is a recurrent phenomenon in those with major affective disorders. Also, because there is a distinct genetic loading in persons with depressive disorder, a family history is vital. Grief is a universal phenomenon, however, and a history of mental illness need not eliminate the possibility that the problem is a simple grieving response.

It is also common to see a mixture between these two processes; a patient may have a major depression *and* be depressed as a response to loss. A person with a propensity to develop a major affective disorder may be more prone to develop a significant degree of depression secondary to a situation involving loss. Although antidepressants may elevate the mood of someone with a major depression, it is unlikely that they are a useful remedy for grief. In fact, the depression seen in grief is not generally treated by medication but through techniques discussed in the next chapter under "Grief Work."

Small Injury—Big Problem

As previously described, severity of injury, apparent disfigurement, and functional disability have been implicated as predictors of long-term adjustment problems after an injury (9). However, patients who experience the injury as a significant narcissistic injury, even if this is not their predominant personality style, can have significant postinjury emotional problems. This may be true even if the injury is relatively minor.

A study at our medical center (10) involved 68 patients between the ages of 18 and 32 years who were hospitalized for more than 1 week with mild or moderate burns. They had adequate social and economic support, and preexisting psychopathology, substance abuse, or medical illness were absent. From this group, 16 patients were identified who were unable to resume social or occupational functions even after months and who were impaired by psychological symptoms related to the injury. These patients were compared to those who did not have any difficulty functioning after the injury. There were no differences between the two groups with respect to age, sex, race, hospital length of stay, agent of injury, circumstances of the accident, or amount of disfigurement.

Those in the group who had problems did develop more sleep disturbances during the hospitalization, and the disrupted sleep continued posthospitalization. This group was also more likely to use regression and displacement as defense mechanisms. People in this group tended to experience the injury as a narcissistic injury and seemed to be more prone to sexual dysfunctions. There were no differences in the amount of psychological treatment the patients received while in the hospital.

In the above study, one prognostic sign, the absence of affective spontaneity, especially shortly before the time of discharge, when pain and medical difficulties were resolved, indicated that a patient with a minor injury might develop emotional problems. In other words, the patients who subsequently developed problems did not join in the bantering humor with staff that is typical at discharge time.

CASE STUDY 1

A 26-year-old woman carpenter sustained second and third degree burn injuries to her upper arm while installing a gas burner. Despite an excellent physical recovery following hospital treatment, she became anxious and depressed and had difficulty sleeping. She had poor appetite and suffered weight loss; she lost interest in herself and her career. She made numerous visits to her plastic surgeon, developed fears of another injury, and became tearful and suicidal. In several visits with the psychiatrist some of her underlying conflicts became apparent. The patient, despite being an attractive, feminine woman, had been the tomboy of the family. Her career in heavy construction was related to her identification with her father; she had been made to feel guilty as a child about this identification. She had suppressed her memory of these issues. The injury, although relatively minor, was experienced as a punishment, and brought to the surface old childhood emotions that made her feel guilty and depressed (10).

Patient Fantasy About Injury

Every patient who sustains an injury will relive the injury and the circumstances related to it in a fantasy. This can occur even when there has been total amnesia about the accident. The victim ponders the details of the accident based on information that has been related, and fills in the gaps. As described below, this is part of the posttraumatic stress response. The actual details of the accident may be reworked and distorted.

As with any physical illness (11), the patient develops a fantasy about the reasons for the accident and the injury. These ideas may fit in with the actual facts of the incident or may be a complete distortion. Even though the patient may recognize the fantasy as "foolish," the fantasy may be personally important and meaningful.

For physical illness and for accidental injuries, the fantasy reflects the basic personality structure of the individual. Understanding this fantasy will usually benefit any psychotherapeutic work in the postinjury period.

The patient frequently questions his or her own role in the accident. This occurs even when the patient had no connection with the cause of the accident. This kind of thinking is almost universal when a child or other loved one is injured or killed in the same accident.

CASE STUDY 2

A 45-year-old man and his family were in an auto accident; the car was hit from the rear. He blamed himself for having neglected to repair the brakes in his car and felt that their condition must have contributed to the accident.

CASE STUDY 3

A high school chemistry teacher was injured in a gas explosion at home. He felt embarrassed and humiliated because he had always stressed safety and caution. He believed that he should have detected the gas leak and that he must have done something wrong that contributed to the accident.

If a person's actions have actually contributed to the injury, there may be great reluctance on the part of that person to discuss such feelings because of the implications to the future legal case. "Hypothetical discussions" may be helpful although the patient will often not be able to discuss his feelings until the case is settled. Sometimes, guilt feelings can be discussed by acknowledging the regret and sorrow that the patient has, but avoiding feelings about culpability.

A patient may experience the accident as a punishment or retribution for past sins, possibly in the form of a religious idea ("God is punishing me") or in a fatalistic view ("I deserve what I got"). Rather than immediately dissuading the patient that this is not the case, it is valuable to first understand why he or she believes such a punishment was deserved. In response to an empathic question, the patient, at this point, may reveal an important understanding that could be useful in subsequent psychological treatment.

CASE STUDY 4

A 55-year-old man was severely injured on his right arm in a printing press accident. He was overheard to say that he "expected something like this to happen sooner or later." An inquiry into the meaning of this statement revealed that he expected it not only because his employer did not maintain the printing press equipment adequately but also because he felt he deserved to be punished for something that had happened more than 35 years ago. As a teenager driving while intoxicated, he had caused an auto accident in which one friend was killed and another was paralyzed.

The same kind of fantasies may also be told by the noninjured who are friends and family of the primary victim. The staff should be alerted to the fact that, during visits to the patient, these individuals may show evidence that they have *also* become psychological casualties of the accident.

When parents are injured, it is particularly important to understand how the child perceives the accident. A 3-year-old who got angry and threw a toy at Mommy the hour before may think he caused his mother's car accident, or a 5-year-old who even fleetingly wished Daddy would go away or be dead may think that somehow her "bad thoughts" caused the fire that burned Daddy. Children may not be able to articulate their fantasies, but might reveal them through play or in drawings.

CASE STUDY 5

A 4-year-old boy whose mother died in a house fire and whose brother was badly injured was seen in the burn center. When he was given crayons and paper, the boy drew a simple house with flames and a stick figure child outside the house holding something that looked like a stick in his hand. When asked about the picture the child explained that the person in the picture was playing with matches and caused the house to be set on fire. The boy in fact had been sleeping when the fire started in the wiring in his house, but he had once played with matches and was punished for the action. He now believed that his transgression caused the death of his mother.

Posttraumatic Stress Symptoms

Quite often, the incident that caused physical injury would be a psychologically traumatic event for almost anyone. Situations such as plane crashes, bizarre accidents, and terrifying fires are clearly out of the range of usual human experience. These events could have been, for example, a serious threat to one's life or physical integrity; a serious threat or harm to one's children, spouse, or other close relatives and friends; sudden destruction of one's home or community; or the witnessing of another person who is seriously injured or has been killed as the result of an accident or physical violence. Being part of such an event in these ways is the first major criteria for posttraumatic stress disorder, as defined in DSM III-R (12).

But even more commonplace situations such as minor accidents, sports injuries, and small burns can bring some psychological symptoms that are part of this disorder. The criteria for DSM III-R can be consulted to determine if a patient has all of the symptoms that officially meet the diagnosis of posttraumatic stress disorder (code no. 309.89) in each category for one month (Table 4.1) (13). However, even when the entire configuration of symptoms and criteria is not present, individual symptoms that are unusually distressing may be present and need to be understood by the treating medical and psychological team.

FLASHBACKS

This general term that most patients understand refers to the reexperiencing of the traumatic event. Patients usually have distressing recollections of the incident that caused their injury. The recollection is often accompanied by anxiety and sometimes by terror. These thoughts may be intrusive and recurrent and in some instances occur completely out of conscious control. Other patients appear to have a need to obsessively ruminate about the traumatic event, often trying to understand or master it. These thoughts can be precipitated by visits of family, friends, and co-workers asking the patient to talk about the accident.

Table 4.1.   Diagnostic Criteria for 309.89 Posttraumatic Stress Disorder[a]

A. The person has experienced an event that is outside the range of usual human experience and that would be markedly distressing to almost anyone, e.g., serious threat to
one's life or physical integrity; serious threat or harm to one's children, spouse, or other
close relatives and friends; sudden destruction of one's home or community; or seeing
another person who has recently been, or is being, seriously injured or killed as a result
of an accident or physical violence.

B. The traumatic event is persistently reexperienced in at least one of the following ways:
   (1) recurrent and intrusive distressing recollections of the event (in young children,
       repetitive play in which themes or aspects of the trauma are expressed)
   (2) recurrent distressing dreams of the event
   (3) sudden acting or feeling as if the traumatic event were recurring (includes a sense
       of reliving the experience, illusions, hallucinations, and dissociative [flashback] epi-
       sodes, even those that occur upon awakening or when intoxicated)
   (4) intense psychological distress at exposure to events that symbolize or resemble an
       aspect of the traumatic event, including anniversaries of the trauma

C. Persistent avoidance of stimuli associated with the trauma or numbing of general
   responsiveness (not present before the trauma), as indicated by at least three of the
   following:
   (1) efforts to avoid thoughts or feelings associated with the trauma
   (2) efforts to avoid activities or situations that arouse recollections of the trauma
   (3) inability to recall an important aspect of the trauma (psychogenic amnesia)
   (4) markedly diminished interest in significant activities (in young children, loss of
       recently acquired developmental skills such as toilet training or language skills)
   (5) feeling of detachment or estrangement from others
   (6) restricted range of affect, e.g., unable to have loving feelings
   (7) sense of a foreshortened future, e.g., does not expect to have a career, marriage,
       or children, or a long life

D. Persistent symptoms of increased arousal (not present before the trauma), as indicated
   by at least two of the following:
   (1) difficulty falling or staying asleep
   (2) irritability or outbursts of anger
   (3) difficulty concentrating
   (4) hypervigilance
   (5) exaggerated startle response
   (6) physiologic reactivity upon exposure to events that symbolize or resemble an
       aspect of the traumatic event (e.g., a woman who was raped in an elevator breaks
       out in a sweat when entering any elevator)

E. Duration of the disturbance (symptoms in B, C, and D) of at least one month.

[a] Reprinted with permission from the *Diagnostic and Statistical Manual of Mental Disorders, Revised.*
Copyright 1987, American Psychiatric Association.

Flashbacks may be quite vivid, with visual and auditory hallucinations, distortions of reality (illusions), and disassociated mood states. The patient feels and acts as if the traumatic event were happening again.

This phenomenon may be precipitated by an organic brain syndrome caused by injury to the central nervous system, by altered metabolic states, or by medication. For example, it would not be unusual for a flashback to occur after a large dosage of narcotic, while waking up from anesthesia or even from normal sleep, or during dressing changes of a burn. The latter situation may cause a flashback not only because of an altered state due to pain medication, but, invariably, because the patient reexperiences actual physical pain.

Also, it is not unusual for an external stimuli such as a news report or the sounds of a fire siren to remind the patient of the event and bring a flashback. Scenes of a television movie may be particularly disturbing to patients.

DREAMS

Individuals may also use the term *flashback* to refer to recurrent, distressing dreams of the traumatic event. These dreams may be typical anxiety dreams, which depict the traumatic event as it actually happened. The dreams may also contain symbolic representations of actual events that are revealed through displacement of the feelings onto other situations or circumstances. Frequently, the patient wakes up in the middle of the dream in an anxious or terrified state. The patient often recalls segments of the dream in great detail, without the usual repression of the dreamer.

This kind of dream may be viewed as a failed attempt to handle anxiety related to the traumatic event and to the underlying conflicts that have been aroused. The repetitive nature of the dream can be understood as an attempt to master the emotions related to the trauma or as a disruption of the functions of the ego.

Close attention to the report of a repetitive dream reveals slight changes in content in each subsequent dream. This appears to reflect the unconscious struggle to master the traumatic experience.

CASE STUDY 6

A 28-year-old man who was injured in an automobile accident had a recurrent dream. In each version, he tried a different method of getting out of the car—crawling to the back, rolling down the window, or opening the door.

Finally, in yet another dream, he broke the rear window and climbed out. In reality, he had done none of these things; the police had rescued him.

NUMBING

Patients who have experienced a psychologically traumatic event may be noted to persistently avoid thoughts or feelings that are associated with the trauma and that might arouse recollections of it. This behavior is similar to the denial and withdrawal described above.

The patient may not be able to recall an important aspect of the trauma. This lack of recall should be distinguished from a head injury with resulting organic mental syndrome and, sometimes, retrograde amnesia starting from the time of the accident and going backward for a variable amount of time. The psychogenic amnesia described here concerns only details of the trauma and will usually be the only apparent memory or cognitive deficit present.

This numbing reaction can include a diminution of interest in activities or a detachment or estrangement from family, friends, and medical staff. The patient shows a restricted range of affect. Emotions of happiness or depression experienced prior to the accident are now muted. This numbing is particularly distressing to family, who find the loved one unable to reciprocate their loving feelings.

Perhaps because the victim of trauma had his or her sense of immortality or invulnerability shattered by the accident, he may feel a sense of foreshortened future. The person will not expect to have an intact job or marriage when released from the hospital, despite reassurances to the contrary. In others, there will be a pessimistic view about marriage, children, and a long life.

INCREASED AROUSAL AND HYPERVIGILANCE

Part of the response to a psychologically traumatic event may be persistent symptoms of increased arousal that were not present before the trauma. Such symptoms may include difficulty falling asleep or staying asleep, irritability or outbursts of anger, difficulty concentrating, hypervigilance, or an exaggerated startle response. An event that symbolizes or resembles an aspect of the trauma may trigger physiological reactions. For example, early in the hospitalization the patient may respond to a nurse who is going to do a painless procedure with the same anxiety that was demonstrated when the staff in the emergency room did a painful procedure.

CASE STUDY 7

A 35-year-old woman survived a single-engine plane crash. In the hospital she became agitated with rapid breathing and perspiration whenever she heard a sound she interpreted as a plane engine.

Course of Psychological Reactions to Burn and Trauma

The reactions to trauma discussed above are time-limited—temporary, usually expected responses of the patient to what has happened. The reactions will change over time. Withdrawal, regression, denial, numbing, depression, anger, and increased arousal usually diminish quickly as the patient makes a physical recovery and can assume increasing independence. Invasive dreams and flashbacks usually decrease in frequency, and fantasies about the injury become integrated with reality. In many patients, all of those symptoms are in remission within 1–2 weeks. In other patients, the symptoms may not completely fade for 1 or 2 months. Occasionally, reactions to burn and trauma recur or can be reactivated several months or even years later due to another trauma or threat. A small number of patients may have full-blown posttraumatic stress disorder.

It is necessary for the treatment team of the trauma and burn patient to be aware of the nature of the patient's psychological response to injury. There is value in reassuring the patient and family that certain responses are an expected part of the patient's normal process of coping with the trauma.

At times, the medical, nursing, and rehabilitation staffs become concerned about a particular patient's response to injury or hospitalization. They may request that the psychiatrist prescribe tranquilizers for vivid flashbacks, antidepressants for normal grief reactions, or sedatives for agitation and angry outbursts. Because they are familiar with the range of normal responses to trauma, the mental health professionals can often show the staff that upsetting behaviors are diminishing in frequency and may resolve entirely without unnecessary medication. However, as described later, psychotropic medication can play a useful role in alleviating some uncomfortable symptoms. Also, specific supportive nursing techniques or psychotherapeutic interventions may help. Some of these are noted in the next chapter. Alternatively, the liaison psychiatrist, mental health nurse, or social worker may have to work on the staff's sense of helplessness in the face of the patient's response.

Personality Types Related to Patient Reaction to Illness

There are many combinations of personality types. By recognizing individuals with a predominant fixed style, staff caring for the patient can better understand patient/staff interactions. Thus, interventions that will decrease patient anxiety and promote psychosocial adaptation to the stress of hospitalization can be appropriately planned.

Kahana and Bibring (14) have described seven basic personality types in terms of psychological reactions to physical illness. These basic personality types have important applicability to burn and trauma patients. These patients do not necessarily have a DSM III-R Axis I diagnosis of major psychiatric illness. Rather, they show a fixed personality style. The descriptions are more similar to the personality diagnosis found on Axis II of the American Psychiatric Association official nomenclature but do not necessarily coincide with these categories.

Following are the categories of personality styles discussed by Kahana and Bibring (14). A case example of each person who has a burn or trauma injury is included along with reports of management interventions.

ORAL PERSONALITY

The oral personality type is a dependent, overdemanding patient who has a great need for personal attention. Following an injury, this need is usually manifested by endless requests for support, interest, and attention from the family and health care providers. A decreased tolerance for frustration, some form of addiction, and an underlying fear of abandonment are common in this group.

CASE STUDY 8

Mr. B. was a 36-year-old man who sustained multiple injuries in a motor vehicle accident. At the time of the accident, he was living with his mother, to whom he was very devoted and who was devoted to him.

While in the critical care unit the nurses became increasingly annoyed as he rang the call bell every few minutes and demanded their almost constant attention. Staff members did not like to go into his room because his requests seemed endless, and leaving the room was next to impossible. Other patients on the unit were more critically injured and needed nursing time.

The patient was seen by a member of the mental health team who set aside a period of time each day to discuss the patient's fears with him and provide him with undivided attention. As the patient's emotional needs became increasingly met by an ongoing therapeutic relationship, he was less in need of constant reassurance from the nurses and other staff members and they viewed the patient in a more positive light.

COMPULSIVE PERSONALITY

Patients who have compulsive personalities are generally self-disciplined and hold a rigid belief system with high expectations for themselves and others. After an injury, they may become very upset by the loss of control over their lives and their inability to maintain strict standards of personal hygiene.

CASE STUDY 9

Mr. C. was a 57-year-old accountant with burns on his arms and hands from a cooking oil fire in his home. He was described by his family as very controlling as well as neat and orderly.

Mr. C. found the need for assistance extremely difficult to tolerate and was in tears several times throughout the day. The comforting words of the staff did little to reassure him and his anxiety continued to escalate.

When this patient was discussed at psychosocial rounds, the psychiatrist, who had seen the patient several times in routine follow-up, discussed with the team the patient's need for control and ways to increase the patient's participation in decision-making and burn care. The patient was given more responsibility for planning his day and the order of his personal hygiene activities. A greater effort was made to explain procedures well in advance and involve the patient in scheduling the order of his daily cares. He was encouraged to focus on keeping a record of his intake and output, his response to pain medication, and his daily schedule of activities. Once the patient felt a degree of control over his situation, his emotional outlook improved considerably.

HYSTERICAL PERSONALITY

Patients reacting in hysterical ways to illness or injury tend to be very dramatic and initially captivating. They may have a tremendous fear of becoming unattractive and subsequently unloved. They may be easily upset and become romantically attached to or have romantic feelings for their caregivers.

CASE STUDY 10

Ms. M., a 26-year-old journalist, accidently amputated her right foot while mowing the lawn with a power mower. While her injury was in itself dramatic enough, she told the story over and over again to anyone who would listen and, with each retelling, added more details. As family and friends tired of the story she sought strangers to talk to and praised continually the attentiveness of a particular male surgical resident who she said was "the only one to have true compassion for me."

While the nurses and resident were initially very happy to support Ms. M., they gradually became more upset with her behavior and responses. They asked the mental health team for assistance in dealing with her. The staff was guided to give the patient positive feedback concerning her competence and performance of required tasks and, at the same time, the patient was encouraged to keep a journal of her emotional responses to her experience. Female nurses were reminded to remain in the room when the favored resident was with the patient to eliminate the ambiguous messages and romantic notions of the patient. The mental health team followed up with the patient to focus on her concerns about her appearance and attractiveness.

MASOCHISTIC PERSONALITY

The patient with a masochistic type personality has frequently had a succession of illnesses or disappointments in life. Such patients may suffer silently, with little regard for their own well-being, because of their need to show concern for others. They may seem to get gratification from reliving the misery of their situation and may even experience the injury as punishment or as expiation for a deep sense of guilt.

CASE STUDY 11

Ms. B. was involved in a car accident that resulted in several facial lacerations and bilateral leg fractures to herself and minor injuries to her 5-year-old daughter. She had been married three times and was recently divorced once again. She reported abandonment by her husband, loss of a job, lack of support from family, and a series of disappointing relationships. Following her injury, she focused all of her attention and concern on her daughter and on the other patients on the unit, insisting that others were much worse off. She rarely asked for pain medications and dismissed the staff's attention. Rather than ask for help she suffered skin breakdown from lying in a bed that had been wet by the spillage of her wash basin during morning cares.

A social worker worked closely with the patient to reinforce the fact that her needs were real and important and to affirm her sense of self-worth. Pain medications were put on an around-the-clock schedule and assessed each day in order to eliminate the patient's need to request relief. Discharge planning involved a visiting nurse and ongoing counseling services that the patient was able to accept initially by focusing on the benefits to her daughter. Gradually, the patient was able to see how her passive acceptance of "one more trouble" fed her underlying sense of guilt.

PARANOID PERSONALITY

Patients reacting according to the paranoid personality type tend to be suspicious, querulous, and potentially litigious. During hospitalization, they may become oversensitive to any type of perceived slight and are suspicious of attempts to help them. They may blame nurses or doctors for their failure to recover more rapidly and report to their families a series of slights or mistreatment.

CASE STUDY 12

Mr. J, a 34-year-old man, came to the burn unit following an industrial accident, in which he was burned on his hands and legs when a chemical was accidently spilled on him. To the embarrassment of his young wife, Mr. J. complained bitterly about his care and about various of the unit's policies. The staff found itself frequently defending the care that this patient received and arguing on behalf of the doctors. Negative feelings about the patient were discussed at psychosocial rounds with the mental health team.

A patient such as this one believes that the statements that he is making are true and will increase his attacks if caregivers attempt to argue against him. Likewise, agreeing with the patient in order to halt his unceasing complaints may only increase his anger by adding credibility to his complaints. The approach with this patient was to acknowledge his beliefs but not to offer an opinion about them. By occasionally asking the patient for his patience with difficult situations he can be steered away from defensiveness and toward a more cooperative mode. As soon as possible, he was taught to do his own dressing changes and allowed to take showers so that he did not need to rely as much on staff that he did not trust. The family was counseled to understand that the patient's complaints had more to do with his fear and sense of helplessness than with his poor care.

SCHIZOID PERSONALITY

The person with a schizoid personality tends to be shy, aloof, remote, and unsociable. The injury of such patients threatens their tenuous psychological equilibrium and their withdrawal will often intensify in proportion to their underlying anxiety.

CASE STUDY 13

Ms. B. was a 42-year-old single woman who was burned in a house fire that involved only herself and left her with deep burns over 50% of her body. As she slowly recovered and was able to be taken out of her room to visit in the dayroom and in the unit, she became more withdrawn and resistive to movement. The staff, assuming that she was depressed about the accident, tried to engage her in conversation and draw her out. Frustrated by their lack of success, staff members turned to the mental health team for help.

When a more thorough psychosocial history of this patient was obtained, it was easy to see that social situations increased the patient's fear of closeness. She was not depressed but anxious about encounters with staff members and other patients. She needed privacy and a quiet, unintrusive approach. She was a patient who never fit comfortably into the social banter of a burn unit but could be helped gradually to increase her ability to relate to people in a limited manner.

NARCISSISTIC PERSONALITY

The narcissistic personality type of patient tends to feel superior and grandiose. These patients want to be powerful and all important and often appear vain and arrogant. Their injury threatens their image of perfection and invulnerability.

CASE STUDY 14

Mr. J. was a successful 30-year-old attorney who had fallen off a ladder while cleaning a gutter at his home on the weekend. In the early phase of hospitalization, he was very cooperative as his open leg fracture was repaired and his collapsed lung healed. However, as his condition improved, he demanded to talk to the doctors more often and resisted the care of house staff and nurses. His demands upset the staff and alienated other patients.

Rather than argue with this patient, the head nurse spoke with him in a calm and matter-of-fact tone and put in place a plan whereby she would speak with the patient each day about his needs. In addition, the attending physician made a point of seeing the patient for a few minutes every day. It was acknowledged by the staff that, since a general personality style is not likely to change, staff energies are conserved by putting in place a plan that accommodates the patient's needs. A few minutes with an "authority" figure may make all the difference in satisfying the narcissistic patient.

Psychological and Psychiatric Symptoms Caused by Drugs

Many commonly used drugs can cause serious psychological and psychiatric symptoms, including depression and even psychotic syndromes that may resemble schizophrenia. These effects may be related to the dosage or can be idiosyncratic. The symptoms that begin while patients are taking a drug usually disappear after the drug is stopped. Some drugs cause symptoms when they are withdrawn, as discussed in the chapter on alcohol and substance abuse.

Table 4.2. Some Drugs That Cause Psychiatric Symptoms[a]

Drug	Reactions	Comments
Acyclovir (Zovirax)	Hallucinations, fearfulness, confusion, insomnia, hyperacusis, paranoia, depression	At high doses, particularly in patients with chronic renal failure
Albuterol (Proventil; Ventolin)	Hallucinations, paranoia	Several reports
Alprazolam (Xanax)	See Benzodiazepines	
Amantadine (Symmetrel[b])	Visual hallucinations, paranoid delusions, nightmares, mania, exacerbation of schizophrenia	Several reports; more frequent in elderly
Aminocaproic acid (Amicar[b])	Acute delirium, hallucinations	Following bolus injection in one patient
Amiodarone (Cordarone)	Delirium, hallucinations	In one patient
Amphetamine-like drugs	Bizarre behavior, hallucinations, paranoia, agitation, anxiety, manic symptoms	Usually with overdose or abuse; can occur with inhaler abuse
	Depression	On withdrawal
Amphotericin B (Fungizone)	Delirium	With IV and intrathecal use
Anabolic steroids	Aggression, mania, depression, psychosis	Several reports
Anticonvulsants	Agitation, confusion, delirium, depression, psychosis, aggression, mania, toxic encephalopathy	Usually with high doses or high plasma concentrations
Antidepressants, tricyclic	Mania or hypomania; delirium, hallucinations, paranoia	Mania or hypomania in about 10% of patients; also after withdrawal
Antihistamines	Anxiety, hallucinations, delirium	Especially with overdosage
Asparaginase (Elspar)	Confusion, depression, paranoia	May occur frequently
Atenolol (Tenormin)	See Beta-adrenergic blockers	
Atropine and anticholinergics	Confusion, memory loss, disorientation, depersonalization, delirium, auditory and visual hallucinations, fear, paranoia, agitation, bizarre behavior	More frequent in elderly and children with high doses; has occurred with transdermal scopolamine
	Sudden incoherent speech, delirium with high fever, flushed dry skin, hallucinations	From eye drops, particularly when mistaken for nose drops
Baclofen (Lioresal[b])	Hallucinations, paranoia, nightmares, mania, depression, anxiety, confusion	Sometimes with treatment, but usually after sudden withdrawal
Barbiturates	Excitement, hyperactivity, visual hallucinations, depression, delirium-tremens-like syndrome	Especially in children and the elderly, or on withdrawal
Belladonna alkaloids	See Atropine and anticholinergics	
Benzodiazepines	Rage, hostility, paranoia, hallucinations, depression, insomnia, nightmares, anterograde amnesia	During treatment or on withdrawal; maybe more common in elderly
Beta-adrenergic blockers	Depression, confusion, nightmares, hallucinations, paranoia, delusions, mania, hyperactivity	With usual doses, including ophthalmic use

Drug	Reaction	Comment
Betaxolol (*Kerlone*)	See Beta-adrenergic blockers	
Bromocriptine (*Parlodel*)	Mania, delusions, hallucinations, paranoia, aggressive behavior, schizophrenic relapse, depression, anxiety	Not dose-related; may persist weeks after stopping drug
Buprenorphine (*Buprenex*)	See Narcotics	
Bupropion (*Wellbutrin*)	Psychosis, hallucinations, agitation, paranoia	In depressed patients; aggravation of symptoms in schizophrenics
Caffeine	Anxiety, confusion, psychotic symptoms	With excessive doses
Captopril (*Capoten*)	Severe anxiety, hallucinations, insomnia, mania	Especially in depressed patients
Carbamazepine (*Tegretol*[b])	See Anticonvulsants	
Cephalosporins	Confusion, disorientation, paranoia, hallucinations	Several reports
Chlorambucil (*Leukeran*)	Hallucinations, lethargy, seizures, stupor, coma	In 5 of 6 patients at high dosage
Chloroprocaine (*Nesacaine*)	See Procaine derivatives	
Chloroquine (*Aralen*[b])	Confusion, delusions, hallucinations	Several reports
Ciprofloxacin (*Cipro*)	Delirium	In one patient
Cimetidine (*Tagamet*)	See Histamine H_2-receptor antagonists	
Clomiphene citrate (*Clomid*[b])	Schizophrenia-like symptoms, paranoia	Two reports
Clonazepam (*Klonopin*)	See Benzodiazepines	
Clonidine (*Catapres*[b])	Delirium, hallucinations, depression	May resolve with continued use
Clorazepate (*Tranxene*[b])	See Benzodiazepines	
Cocaine	Anxiety, agitation, psychosis	Can occur with topical use
Codeine	See Narcotics	
Contraceptives, oral	Depression	In 15% in one study
Corticosteroids, (prednisone, cortisone, ACTH, others)	Mania, depression, confusion, paranoia, hallucinations, catatonia	Especially with high doses; can occur on withdrawal or with inhalation
Cyclobenzaprine (*Flexeril*[b])	Mania, hyperactivity, psychosis	In three patients
Cyclopentolate (*Cyclogyl*)	See Atropine and anticholinergics	
Cycloserine (*Seromycin*[b])	Anxiety, depression, confusion, psychosis	Common
Cyclosporine (*Sandimmune*)	Hallucinations; mania	Each in one patient
Dapsone	Insomnia, agitation, hallucinations, mania, depression	Several reports; may occur even with low doses
Deet (*Off*[b])	Toxic encephalopathy, mania, hallucinations	With excessive or prolonged use, particularly in infants and children
Nifedipine (*Procardia; Adalat*)	Irritability, agitation, panic, belligerence, depression	Several reports
Niridazole (*Ambilhar*)	Confusion, hallucinations, mania, suicide	More likely with higher doses
Nonsteroidal anti-inflammatory drugs	Paranoia, depression, inability to concentrate, anxiety, confusion, hallucinations, hostility	Not reported with all drugs in this class
Norfloxacin (*Noroxin*)	Depression; anxiety	Anxiety in one patient
Oxandrolone	See Anabolic steroids	
Oxymetazoline (*Afrin*[b])	Hallucinations, anxiety, insomnia	With nasal decongestants in children

Table 4.2. (Continued)ᵃ

Drug	Reactions	Comments
Oxymetholone (Anadrol)	See Anabolic steroids	
Pargyline (Eutonyl)	Manic psychosis	In one patient
Penicillin G Procaine	See Procaine derivatives	
Pentazocine (Talwin)	See Narcotics	
Pergolide (Permax)	Hallucinations, paranoia, confusion; anxiety; depression	On withdrawal
Phenelzine (Nardil)	Paranoia, delusions, fear, mania, rage	Mania or hypomania in about 10% of depressed patients
Phenmetrazine (Preludin)	See Amphetamine-like drugs	
Phentermine (Fastinᵇ)	See Amphetamine-like drugs	
Phenylephrine (Neo-Synephrineᵇ)	Depression, hallucinations, paranoia	Overuse of nasal spray
Phenylpropanolamine (Dexatrimᵇ)	See Amphetamine-like drugs	
Phenytoin (Dilantinᵇ)	See Anticonvulsants	
Podophyllin	Delirium, paranoia, bizarre behavior	Oral use in child, topical in 2 adults
Polythiazide (Renese)	Depression	In two patients after 2 weeks' use
Prazosin (Minipressᵇ)	Hallucinations, depression, paranoia	In four patients; two had renal failure
Primidone (Mysolineᵇ)	See Anticonvulsants	
Procainamide (Pronestylᵇ)	See Procaine derivatives	
Procaine derivatives	Terror, confusion, psychosis, agitation, bizarre behavior, depression, panic	Many reports, especially with Penicillin G Procaine
Procarbazine (Matulane)	Mania	In one patient
Promethazine (Phenerganᵇ)	Hallucinations, terror	In two children
Propoxyphene (Darvonᵇ)	See Narcotics	
Propranolol (Inderalᵇ)	See Beta-adrenergic blockers	
Pseudoephedrine (in Actifed)	Hallucinations, paranoia	Reported with usual dosage in children and with overuse in one adult
Quinacrine (Atabrine)	Mania, paranoia, anxiety, hallucinations, delirium	More common with high doses
Quinidine	Confusion, agitation, psychosis	Usually dose-related
Ranitidine (Zantac)	See Histamine H₂-receptor antagonists	
Reserpine (Serpasilᵇ)	Depression, nightmares	Common with >0.5 mg/day
Salicylates	Agitation, confusion, hallucinations, paranoia	Chronic intoxication
Scopolamine (Hyoscineᵇ)	See Atropine and anticholinergics	
Sulindac (Clinoril)	See Nonsteroidal anti-inflammatory drugs	

Theophylline	Withdrawal, mutism, hyperactivity; anxiety; mania	Usually with high serum concentrations
Thiabendazole (Mintezol)	Psychic disturbances	Occasional
Thyroid hormones	Mania, depression, hallucinations, paranoia	Initial doses in susceptible patients
Timolol (Timoptic[b])	See Beta-adrenergic blockers	
Tobramycin (Nebcin)	Delirium, hallucinations, agitation	In one 66-year-old patient
Tocainide (Tonocard)	See Procaine derivatives	
Tranylcypromine (Parnate)	Mania or hypomania	In about 10% of depressed patients
Trazodone (Desyrel[b])	Delirium, hallucinations, paranoia, mania	Several reports
Triazolam (Halcion)	See Benzodiazepines	
Trichlormethiazide (Naqua[b])	Depression; suicidal ideation	In two patients after 2–3 months' use
Trihexyphenidyl (Artane[b])	See Atropine and anticholinergics	
Trimethoprim-sulfamethoxazole (Bactrim[b])	Psychosis; depression, disorientation	Few reports
Valproic acid (Depakene[b])	See Anticonvulsants	
Verapamil (Isoptin; Calan[b])	Auditory, visual and tactile hallucinations	In one woman
Vincristine (Oncovin[b])	Hallucinations	Less than 5% of patients; high doses
Zidovudine (Retrovir)	Mania with paranoia, hallucinations	Reported in two patients

[a] Reprinted with permission from *The Medical Letter on Drugs and Therapeutics* (15).
[b] Also available with other brands or generically.

Patients who suffer a sudden unexpected burn or trauma injury may have been taking drugs that may or may not be continued after they enter the hospital. During the course of treatment, new drugs may be introduced by a variety of specialists caring for the patient. Whenever patients on medication have a changed mental status or new psychological or psychiatric symptoms, the role of the drug in producing the symptoms should be considered.

The Medical Letter on Drugs and Therapeutics has produced a useful table in this regard (15) (see Table 4.2.).

References

1. Mieszala P. Postburn psychological adaptation: an overview. Crit Care Q 1978;93–111.
2. Engel GI, Reichsman F. Spontaneous and experimentally induced depression in an infant with a gastric fistula: a contribution to the problem of depression. J Am Psychoanal Assoc 1956;4:428.
3. Dubovsky SL. The psychophysiology of health, illness and stress. In: Simons RC, Pardes H, eds. Understanding human behavior in health and illness. Baltimore: Williams & Wilkins. 2nd ed. 1981:90.
4. Blumenfield M, Thompson TL. The psychological reactions to physical illness. In: Simons RC, Pardes H, eds. Understanding human behavior in health and illness. 2nd ed. Baltimore: Williams & Wilkins, 1981.
5. Averill JR. Anger and aggression: an essay on emotion. New York: Springer, 1982.
6. Strain JJ. Psychological intervention in medical practice. New York: Appleton-Century-Crofts, 1978.
7. Strain JJ, Grossman S. Psychological reaction to medical illness and hospitalization. In: Strain JJ, Grossman S, eds. Psychological care of the medically ill: a primer in liaison psychiatry. New York: Appleton-Century- Crofts, 1975.
8. Freud S. Mourning and melancholia. Standard ed. 1917;14: 239–258.
9. Andreasen NJC, Norris AS, Hartford CE. Incidence of long-term psychiatric complication in severely burned adults. Ann Surg 1971;174:785–793.
10. Blumenfield M, Reddish PM. Identification of psychologic impairment in patients with mild-moderate thermal injury. Small burn, big problem. Gen Hosp Psychiatry 1987;9:142–146.
11. Blumenfield M. Fantasies about physical illness. Psychother Psychosom 1983;39:171–179.
12. Diagnostic and statistical manual of mental disorders. DSM III-R. 3rd ed. revised. Washington: American Psychiatric Association, 1987:250.
13. Diagnostic and statistical manual of mental disorders. DSM III-R. 3rd ed. revised. Washington: American Psychiatric Association, 1987.
14. Bibring GL, Kahana RJ. Lectures in medical psychology. New York: International Universities Press, 1968:246.
15. Drugs that cause psychiatric symptoms. Med Lett Drugs Ther 1989;31:113–116.

Psychological Interventions

Ideally, all hospital settings where burn and trauma patients are treated should have a close working relationship with at least one mental health professional who sees the patient early in the course of hospitalization. Patients vary in readiness and need for psychological intervention. There should be regular "rounds" or follow-up to determine if patients need such work. The medical and nursing staff who are involved with the patient daily, and sometimes on a minute-to-minute basis, can alert the mental health professional of any change in mental status or need for intervention.

For all patients, the very first need is physical comfort. As pointed out in Chapter 1, pain issues must be considered before any psychotherapeutic approach is begun. Once pain is under control, the following psychological interventions may be appropriate.

Grief Work

Every patient who has suffered a burn or traumatic injury has sustained a loss. There may be a loss of function, role, independence, or of the sense of safety in the world. The patient may have lost his home or possessions. Even more significantly, loved ones may have died.

While the nature of the loss may seem self-evident, this is not always the case. Before the patient's grieving process can be understood, there needs to be a thorough assessment of what the patient believes he has lost. Often, things are not what they seem.

CASE STUDY 1

A 26-year-old artist experienced the traumatic amputation of her dominant arm in an automobile accident. By the end of the first week of hospitalization, the medical and nursing staff voiced concern that the woman had expressed no sadness about being unable to paint again. Talking to the clinical nurse specialist, the patient revealed that she really had wanted to pursue another career even before the accident. But she related that she was devastated by the thought that she would never be able to embrace the baby she dreamed of having one day.

There are other examples revealing that the significance of the loss may not be apparent. For example, the death of a distant great aunt was especially traumatic for a young adult; the aunt had been an important role model. A person whose house is destroyed by fire may focus on personal photographs of deceased parents rather than on financial loss. The loss of a family pet may not be fully appreciated. One patient described such a loss: "That dog was the only living creature that accepted me exactly as I am."

Not only might the true significance or meaning of a loss be unapparent to the outside observer, but the grieving person may also need help to clarify the object of his or her grief. A person escaping from a motor vehicle accident with a minor injury requiring only 3 or 4 days of hospitalization may be unusually distraught. The loss of invulnerability or the sense of safety in the world can trigger a full-blown grief response that confuses the patient until he is helped to understand this loss.

Grieving is a natural process. *Grief work* is a term applied to this activity: both the obvious process of mourning and the intrapsychic readjustment necessary for the resolution of loss (1). Threatened loss can trigger an anticipatory grief that is as powerful as the grief of an actual loss. Grief work takes time and cannot be hurried. One of the biggest mistakes well-meaning professionals and friends make is to try to turn off the emotions associated with loss or to hurry the painful process. There is no timetable that works for everyone, although various authors have described the grief response as a series of stages.

STAGES OF GRIEF WORK

In her books on death and dying (2–4), Kubler-Ross discusses five stages of grief—denial, bargaining, anger, depression, and acceptance. Not every person goes through all the stages, and the stages may not be in any special order. Sometimes it is impossible to differentiate between the stages; individuals do not move neatly from one to another.

Westberg, in *Good Grief*, emphasizes that grief has a beginning, middle, and end (5). He has delineated the following 10 stages of recovery from loss and has highlighted the growth aspects of this process toward acceptance:

1. Shock

2. Emotional expression
3. Depression
4. Physical symptoms (somatization of pain)
5. Panic (can think of nothing else)
6. Guilt about the loss
7. Anger and resentment (at God, a loved one, the doctor, the unfairness of life)
8. Resistance to returning (keeping the memory alive)
9. Hope (for a better and less painful time to come)
10. Reality affirmation—acknowledging one can never return to being one's "old self."

FACILITATING GRIEF WORK

However, the stages of grief are defined, the work of grief goes on and can be facilitated for the burn or trauma patient in the following ways.

Acknowledge the Loss

The mental health professional can prompt the patient to look at losses by bringing up the subject that family and others often avoid. Once the loss is out in the open, most patients are more than willing to talk about it, even if they show initial resistance. A few questions or a simple statement such as, "This must have been a very painful loss for you" often promotes an outpouring of emotion that the listener should be prepared to hear.

Allow the Person to Be With the Pain

A caregiver may often have the erroneous notion that somehow he can "save" the bereaved from the pain they are experiencing. Rationalizations about the good that will come of the loss or "positive" aspects of the loss are often pointed out in an attempt to comfort the person in emotional pain. The words may help the *caregiver* feel better, but the pain of loss is not eliminated by words and, more often, the unspoken message is "I have heard enough of your sad woes so let's talk about something more upbeat."

Far more helpful words to the grieving person early in grief work are "I can see you are in a great deal of pain. Tell me more about what that feels like." Such encouraging words as "A time will gradually come when the pain will not be so intense or so ever-present" are appropriate *after* the person has had ample time to express feelings. Even when time is limited, the person experiencing loss needs to feel that the listener or facilitator can bear to hear the full power of his emotions while he is reminiscing.

Affirm the Individual's Experience As Real and Part of Normal Grief

A common comment from a grieving person is "I feel like I am going crazy." Such a comment obviously needs further exploration. Most of the time the explanation is well within the typical grief response. Somatization, preoccupation with the image of the deceased or lost object, guilt, hostility, and loss of normal patterns of conduct are all anticipated parts of a normal grief reaction (6). This is a time to sanction mourning and to allow self-centeredness.

Provide Assurance by Exploring Past Coping Patterns

Since loss may feel unbearable, it is important to help mourners see that they have gone through difficult times in the past. Ask questions such as "What is the most difficult thing you ever went through in the past?" and "How did you manage to get through that difficult time?" Also asking "Whom can you depend on to help you through this?" can give important clues to both the person experiencing the loss and the grief facilitator. This step also yields important data for an assessment of other losses and possible complicating stressors. The cumulative effects of multiple losses without recuperation can be particularly devastating. The pain of previous losses not fully experienced may be rekindled.

MONITORING DANGER SIGNALS

The signals that a grieving person is not handling loss in a healthy way follow (7).

Persistent Thought About Self-Destruction

Although such comments as "I'll never be able to go on without him (or her)" are not unusual, any suicidal ideas must be taken seriously.

Failure to Provide for Basic Survival Needs

Although it is certainly commonplace to forget to eat and to find sleep difficult, the persistent loss of appetite and/or sleep disturbances signal a potentially serious problem.

Persistent Mourning or Long-term Depression

More significant than the length of the mourning process is whether a progression can be observed. Is the grieving person less preoccupied with the loss? More able to invest energies in interests? Or are the symptoms of distress the same or worse over many months or years?

Abuse of Controlling Substances Such As Drugs or Alcohol

Drugs and alcohol can produce temporary numbing from the pain of grief but, in fact, retard the process of recovery. They can also lead to more serious problems.

Recurrence of Mental Illness

Although many persons with serious mental illnesses are surprising in their ability to go through normal grief and mourning, the added stress can be too much for persons already in a precarious balance.

In the presence of any of the above danger signals, a more formal psychiatric evaluation of the patient should be done by a mental health professional and appropriate help should be offered.

EDUCATING PATIENTS AND FAMILIES ABOUT THE NORMALCY OF LOSS, GRIEF, AND MOURNING, AND THE RESOURCES FOR COPING

A good portion of the hospitalized burn or trauma patient's grief work will most likely be continued after the patient is discharged from the acute care facility. Even if a patient appears to be handling his losses while in the hospital, discharge will likely bring about a new adjustment and a new phase of grief work. This should be anticipated prior to discharge in discussion with patients and families, when appropriate referrals to resources in the community can be made.

Even small children have a grief response to loss. In fact, the most significant loss for the child who is burned or sustains a traumatic injury may be the temporary loss of mother and/or father. The separation brought by hospitalization can be very difficult for the child (and parent), and all the responses associated with grief are expected. Frequently, children strike out angrily at Mom and Dad for what they perceive as abandonment. Obviously, the staff wants to allow as much parent contact as possible for children, but loss of familiar surroundings and routines still exists. While children cannot necessarily verbalize their feelings, they often act feelings out through play or new behavior patterns. Play therapy and the use of a child psychiatric consultation should be considered for the youngster who shows significant distress.

Treatment of Regression

One of the most common behaviors noted among burn and trauma patients is regression. Overwhelmed by the many physical and psychological discomforts, a patient may attempt to return to the "good feelings" of a previous time in his life through regression. Some common examples follow.

CASE HISTORIES

CASE 1

A 26-year-old man who was driving while intoxicated hit a stone pillar at the end of his driveway. He suffered a chest contusion, bilateral compound fractures of the lower extremities, and numerous facial lacerations. After six days in the intensive care unit, with both legs in traction, he could be heard crying and making excessive demands on the nurses. He whined for what he wanted and pouted when his needs were not gratified. When his young wife visited he asked her to feed him, and when his mother was present he asked her to speak to the doctors on his behalf. Prior to the injuries, the patient had been a competent, fiercely independent Wall Street analyst.

CASE 2

A 39-year-old woman was in a house fire that caused the death of her 42-year-old husband and one of her three children. She suffered a significant inhalation injury requiring two weeks on a respirator to heal her lungs. In addition, she sustained second and third degree burns over her arms, chest, back, and face—amounting to 35% of her total body surface area. After the patient had finally been extubated and had undergone three debridement and grafting procedures, she became incontinent of urine and stool. She would not even call the nurse to be cleaned up. One night she was found sucking her thumb while sleeping.

CASE 3

A bright, 6-year-old boy was scalded when a coffee urn overturned and spilled on his legs. He sustained burns over 50% of his lower body. After several weeks of immobility, when the time was appropriate to begin walking, the young patient denied an ability to walk and insisted that the best he could do was crawl. For several days he moved about on his hands and knees and cried whenever staff attempted to get him to an upright position.

All three cases above illustrate a regressed clinical presentation. Family members may be shocked to see such behavior and even staff members may have very negative reactions to regression. Handling regression in the injured patient is difficult. Some guiding principles follow.

GUIDELINES

1. Examine caregiver responses first. The staff often view the regressed behavior of a patient as manipulative, and they respond angrily. It may be especially difficult for the staff to deal with the behavior when a patient is male because of societal expectations that men be strong and able to tolerate pain. Labels of "wimp" signal rejection on the part of the staff. Once staff members see that they are negatively "hooked" and are responding to the regressed behavior, as pointed out by the mental health professional working with the staff, they can begin to problem solve and work together with a plan to cope with the behavior until the patient is able to return to higher levels of functioning.

2. Recognize the behavior for what it is—a coping mechanism. Punishment and shaming are never appropriate responses; they do nothing to help the patient meet the need for comforting, safety, or nurturing.

3. Determine whether the behavior interferes with the goals at hand. Whining alone does not interfere with recovery, and will probably disappear quicker when given little attention. But the injured patient with healed hands who still wants to be fed will harm himself or herself if regressed behavior is allowed to continue. A child might benefit from an explanation of the need for the exercise of feeding, and might be offered a substitute form of emotional gratification, such as being read to while feeding. In other instances, daily activity schedules planned with patient and staff together and written down might be useful. Behavior modification techniques, with rewards for achieved goals, are effective with some patients.

4. Develop a consistent plan for handling the regressed behavior. Help significant family members and friends play a part in the plan. Often, the family needs to spend considerable time with the mental health team to understand the regressed behavior and to see their roles in enabling the patient to move from this mode of coping. Without intervention by mental health professionals, family members may spend considerable energy feuding over the proper way to approach the patient.

5. Be clear with the patient and family about what is expected of them. The unspoken expectation of health care providers is that the patient will be able to regress enough to tolerate having things done to him and yet be independent enough to assume some responsibility for recovery. There is no guarantee that the patient and the care-giving team will view the desired level of regression equally, and there is a constant need for dialogue between staff and patient about what is expected.

6. Acknowledge the relinquishment of regressed behavior without ridiculing how a patient "used to behave." In time, many patients will laugh at themselves and at how they coped, but others will hang on to the memory of that period as a painful time of feeling very needy and not receiving much relief or understanding.

FOLLOW-UP OF CASE HISTORIES

The following discussions of mental health team interventions in the three cases presented above helps illustrate a therapeutic approach to the problems of regression:

CASE 1

The psychiatric clinical nurse specialist met with the patient's wife and mother to discuss the patient's behavior and to enlist their cooperation in a plan. Their feelings of frustration at watching the patient regress were recognized and their ideas were incorporated into a plan. Later, when the patient was approached, it was explained to him that the family members were united in an effort to work with the patient toward independence while at the same time working to increase the sense of safety and confidence of the patient. The patient was given individual supportive sessions to deal with his unresolved sense of guilt about the accident.

CASE 2

At the weekly psychosocial rounds the psychiatrist and clinical nurse specialist brought up the issue of the patient's regression. Staff members were invited to share their negative feelings. The magnitude of the loss suffered by this patient was discussed and a plan was put in place that would actually increase the care of the patient for a short time—to support her regression. After 2 days of a full dose of being cared for, the patient's former level of functioning began to return. The patient then had several individual psychotherapy sessions to help her deal with her grief.

CASE 3

The mental health team met with the boy's parents to discuss his regressed behavior. The parents agreed to participate in a plan to advance the patient toward ambulation progressively. Then, the parents and the mental health team, as well as some of the nursing staff, met with the patient. A behavior modification plan with rewards in terms of television time worked well. A written contract and a chart with colorful stickers were placed in the child's room and used to mark his progress.

OTHER APPROACHES TO REGRESSION

An interesting study by Tempereau and others (8) looks at two forms of regressed behavior and the influence of the spouse and significant others in handling these regressions. These authors distinguish between *dependent* and *primitive regression*. The former refers to immature, dependent behavior, such as crying, tantrums, and rebellion, and the latter refers, for example, to "the surly withdrawal reminiscent of a wounded animal and [which is] characterized by sullen withdrawal and persistent molestation of the wounds." In the study, dependent regression was more common in persons with a clearly defined social network, and primitive regression was more often seen in loners, those with individualistic behavior patterns (such as entrepreneurs and executives) and without a structured social support network.

Another significant finding in this study (8) concerns the spouse's response to the patient's dependency needs. When the response is uncharacteristic (the husband who usually gives a "Buck up!" response to whining from his wife suddenly becomes sympathetic), the patient interprets the behavior as abandonment. This suggests that the patient requires the consistency of former responses from a significant other in order to feel safe and able to cope with regression.

In another article, Carnes points out the need to thoroughly assess a patient's dependency status prior to the trauma as well as to obtain a thorough history of how the patient has coped in the past (9). With the elderly and with children in particular, it is essential to know a baseline level of functioning so that realistic goals can be set for the present circumstances.

The good news about regressive behavior is that, while it can be vexing for staff and family members, it is usually time limited. When a patient no longer feels threatened he is ready to move on to other forms of coping.

Expressive and Abreactive Techniques

In this basic psychotherapeutic approach, previously unexpressed feelings are released, often in the form of emotionally charged verbalizations.

Verbalization is an essential part of the technique used to assist a patient with grieving. The patient talks with a full range of emotions—love, hate, anger—about a lost object.

Trauma patients usually have a need to relive the details of the traumatic event. They may try to understand exactly what happened. The patient goes over details numerous times and speculates on possible causes of unexplained details. Alternative actions that could have been taken are pondered. In this recapitulation, emotions may be left out entirely or hidden.

Yet there are many patients who have clear needs to reexperience or relive all the *emotions* connected with an accident. Self-blame and guilt may be part of these ruminations. At this point, abreaction of emotion is helpful without interpretive work.

Patients are usually receptive when they are encouraged to talk out feelings. They express sadness with tears and crying. They will talk about their worry and concern for the present and future. Some of this talk may be quite realistic or it may be exaggerated and obsessional.

The listener who facilitates the patient's expression and abreaction does not necessarily have to be a skillful therapist. Sometimes the treating surgeon, nurse, or occupational therapist can fulfill the important role of listener. The staff must realize that the process of facilitating verbalization is often repetitive. At times it is provocative. The listener requires a certain degree of empathy to put himself in the patient's place and to have some degree of understanding of what the patient must be feeling. The patient's verbalization can be encouraged by responses such as, "I can see how scared you must have been." It is more important to allow patients to express their thoughts and feelings than it is to constantly provide reassurance. Family and friends usually take the reassuring role, but may not want to hear the expression of painful emotions. Corrections of gross reality distortions may be offered if information is readily available, but the patient may not be ready to hear them because of his or her psychological needs at that time.

Expression and abreaction may be the most important therapy the patient can go through during the early stages after an injury. Experienced psychotherapists are able to make judgments about the timing of further interventions and interpretations.

Utilizing the Meaning of the "Brush with Death" To Effect Change

Many patients who have sustained a serious injury requiring hospitalization view the experience as a "brush with death." In some cases, there is be no doubt that loss of life was barely averted by a quirk of fate. Even in circumstances where the injury was nonlife-threatening, it does not take much imagination to realize that with slightly different circumstances, the person would have been killed.

Certainly, with high-speed highways and airplane travel, everyone is only a few seconds away from catastrophe. When a person has a close personal encounter with disaster, in either an individual accident or a mass casualty, the normal denial of mortality is breached. Under these circumstances, the usual psychological defenses that enable a person to block out thoughts about his own death are now lowered.

In many, this lowering of defenses brings the intensification of anxiety previously discussed. It also brings a regression: more vulnerable, childlike feelings and the wish to be cared for by parental figures and parental substitutes. There is a tendency to "take stock." When the sense of immortality characteristic of youth is lifted, there is opportunity and motivation for an honest self-assessment. This is not dissimilar to what happens when a person goes through a "midlife crisis." In such a crisis, a person believes he or she has a last chance to make important changes in life. In such a situation, a person may be mobilized to act and make changes in the marital relationship, or take such actions as buying a coveted sports car or desired jewelry or choosing a new career.

A hospitalized trauma patient who is integrating a brush with death may also go through this midlife crisis. This occurs regardless of the person's age. The patient may begin to plan changes for the future and is often receptive to a psychotherapeutic intervention allowing him or her to sort things out mentally. Sometimes, a person who never would have considered any form of psychotherapy is suddenly glad to have someone with whom he or she can talk.

Asking the patient "How has this event [accident, injury] changed your life?" can be a good entry into the patient's thought process on this topic. The patient's initial response will include statements concerning the nature of the accident: "I will always follow safety rules in the future" or, "I will never drive a small car again." Other statements such as, "I will never drink again" may provide an opportunity to assist the patient, make a referral to an alcohol rehab program, or begin to discuss underlying reasons for such a problem. Other self-assessments such as, "I realize I had better change my life before it is too late" can lead to further clarifications of the meaning of the discontent the patient feels. The desire to continue this process may lead to a referral for outpatient psychotherapy.

Working with the Patient's Fantasy About the Accident

A patient usually has his own idea about the cause of the injury. Even if the actual facts are not known, the patient ultimately forms a very personal theory about the event.

It may be a very important part of any psychological evaluation and intervention to explore this fantasy. In it lie the explanations for the guilt and self-recriminations. Often, these feelings go far beyond the actual event. The patient struggles with self-blame and with the reason why he or she happened to be in a particular job or relationship. The patient may say that had he or she not been in this situation, the accident would not have happened.

Still others relate to the guilt as if it were a punishment by God or some higher force, or an act of fate. Some ideas that the patient brings up in this regard may reflect significant depressive feelings. As previously described, when a positive relationship with the patient has developed, a persistent inquiry can be made to uncover the patient's fantasy about the source of such guilt (10). At this point, the hospitalized patient is likely to be in a psychologically regressed state, with the usual psychological defenses working at less than full capacity.

Often, the fantasy about why the accident occurred is a function of the patient's psychodynamic personality structure. The dependent, depressive patient speaks about a sense of inadequacy and a poor sense of self-worth. The fantasies of some may reflect the expectation of being punished for earlier deeds for which they harbor guilt, or, for example, for not being good spouses. Patients whose predominant personal theme is the competitive or oedipal one will also reflect these thoughts in their personal fantasies describing the reason for their accidents.

The information obtained from this inquiry into the patient's fantasy is helpful in preliminary psychotherapeutic work with the patient. On a superficial level, obviously incorrect facts about the accident can easily be corrected—"The police determined that the skid marks showed that your vehicle was not in the the wrong lane." Any psychodynamic determinant revealed in the fantasy can be helpful in formulating an intervention for some type of therapy, as described below.

The obsessive patient may not be able to make up his or her mind concerning the fantasy. In a similar vein, a patient thinking in a concrete manner might not allow himself or herself to consider any feelings underlying the actual event as he or she knows it. Some patients find it difficult to have any fantasies whatsoever. Such information is always useful in subsequent psychotherapeutic work with patients.

Psychotherapeutic Approach to Anger

A simple inquiry often allows a patient to express emotions that were on the surface, sometimes ready to explode. When such feelings gradually emerge in the course of discussions with the staff or with the psychotherapist, it is usually appropriate to acknowledge them with statements such as, "I understand how at times you get very angry and frustrated." For most people, the very fact of being understood can be comforting and supportive. There is usually no immediate need to redirect the anger or to talk the patient out of any feelings he has.

Family members and friends are often uncomfortable with emotions of anger and depression (as will be discussed below), and they, therefore, try to divert the patient from these emotions or do not listen to such discussions. On the other hand, the frustrated and angry feelings of a family member can sometimes fuel the emotions of the patient. The discussion between an attorney and the patient can affect the patient's emotions. Angry feelings may be channeled and defused as plans for retribution are being made or, instead, these emotions may be intensified.

Often, the patient desires an opportunity to express and abreact angry feelings. This can be handled by the regular nursing staff, although at times it may be advisable for a psychotherapist to talk with the patient about his or her feelings. Such a person should meet regularly with the patient even if the visits are brief. Meeting a couple of times a week and establishing a regular relationship can be useful in letting the patient know there is a "safe place" for anger—an opportunity to talk to someone who, unlike family, does not need to be protected from his or her feelings.

Most of the patient's anger is directed outward, toward external factors that caused the accident—the driver of the other vehicle, the co-worker, the employer, the manufacturer of faulty equipment, the government regulations, the insurance company. The patient expresses frustration about missing work, being in traction, feeling pain, prolonged hospitalization.

At times, the patient also directs anger at the hospital staff for reasons such as delay in their administration of medication or delay in their answering calls; transportation errors, perceived rough handling, visits by medical staff that are considered to be too brief, poor communication by staff. Usually, such expressions are muted; the patient has a natural reluctance to antagonize the medical and nursing staff on whom he is so dependent. It can be particularly useful to help the patient acknowledge such feelings and, by doing so, assure him or her that patient care is not threatened by having and expressing such feelings.

DISPLACED ANGER

At times, the patient's anger gets out of control. The family members who are objects of this anger can be brutally antagonized. Old conflicts and disagreements are rekindled without any apparent reason. The patient also expresses hostility toward the medical and nursing staffs. Small grievances escalate into angry and provocative statements. The patient does not comply with treatment and refuses medications and procedures. Noncompliance is one of the few acting-out behaviors available to the hospitalized patient. Even the most enlightened medical and nursing staffs can be provoked. A typically busy and harried trauma or burn team may find itself becoming antagonistic toward a particular patient in these circumstances. Family and friends withdraw, feeling hurt and antagonized.

All of the pillars of support for this angry trauma or burn patient may become completely alienated from him or her in a short time. This situation is a potentially dangerous situation for everyone involved, particularly the patient. The medical and surgical staffs cannot provide optimal care if they are antagonized and pushed away. Important observations may not be made as frequently as they should. Decisions for necessary procedures may be delayed and even avoided if the patient refuses care. The ultimate refusal occurs when the patient leaves the hospital before treatment has been completed.

Hopefully, before this situation escalates, a psychiatric consultation can be obtained. The differential diagnosis mentioned earlier needs to be considered. The use of tranquilizers for underlying disorders or for short-term relief may be helpful. However, this kind of situation may turn out to be one where the patient's anger is being displaced toward external objects. Unlike the earlier examples of patient anger requiring only an empathic acknowledgment, a delicate interpretation is now in order. Once the situation is understood, the nature of the interpretation becomes quite clear, but its execution requires the most skillful psychotherapist available.

Patients, in reality, are angry at themselves. They are angry about their own role, real or imaginary, in the accident and angry for not having avoided the entire situation. This may include a deep-seated anger for having a certain job or life-style, certain current relationships, or anything else connected to the accident. Patients are angry at themselves for not recovering fast enough, for needing pain medication, for not tolerating the hospitalization. These feelings are mostly unconscious and unacceptable to the patient, and this is why they are displaced onto external objects, such as staff and family. Sometimes there are hidden, unacceptable angry feelings directed at a person the patient believes contributed to the accident or to the current situation. Many of these feelings are unacceptable, originating from anger at one's self, as described above.

Any psychological insight interpretation must be made in the context of a good therapeutic relationship. The patient must like and trust the therapist who makes such an interpretation and have an underlying positive transference (feelings based on earlier childhood relationships) toward the therapist.

In this setting, the therapist must decide whether to attempt to diffuse the troublesome, angry emotions by interpreting their true nature. If this is done, the interpretation from the trusted therapist might be, "While you are blaming the doctors for not recovering fast enough, I think you are really mad at *yourself* for the accident that put you in the hospital."

Although this kind of interpretation is usually very successful in dealing with displaced anger, it can be expected to lead to an intensification of depressed feelings. The defense against inward directed hostility is taken away, and anger that had been directed outward is now directed inward. This can lead to a profound depression and even to suicidal ideation. The decision to take such an interpretive approach should therefore not be taken lightly. The decision is made when the displaced anger threatens to bring harm to the patient through a disruption of necessary medical/surgical care and/or crucial social support. Such an interpretative approach is a calculated risk that the therapist takes, and is not unlike decisions that are made in the operating room when two therapeutic approaches have potential danger. Obviously, if depression and suicidal behavior are anticipated, appropriate precautions must be taken.

There are psychotherapeutic support techniques that can be added at this point, including the use of the transference relationship by the therapist to show the patient particular respect and to praise him or her for acknowledging true feelings.

Another approach is to attempt to make a less than exact interpretation in instances that suggest anger toward an intermediary object. For example, in attempting to diffuse displaced anger directed toward the medical staff, the interpretation might deal with anger at the "accident" or at the "other party." An interpretation might be: "While you are expressing all this anger at the head nurse for asking you to do various things, I think you are really furious at your employers who made you work the extra hours on the day that you were injured." This approach is not usually as successful as acknowledging the underlying self-directed feelings.

Psychodynamic Life Narrative Treatment Approach

Viedermann and Perry have suggested an insight oriented psychotherapeutic technique to treat depression in the physically ill (11). They attempt to make a clear distinction between the approach to grief and the approach to depression. They suggest that grieving patients need empathic understanding to facilitate the work of mourning. As previously discussed, therapists working with such patients need to convey to them that the experience of intense and painful feelings is a "normal" part of the process of adaptation to loss. The therapist working with the depressed patient does not facilitate a normal process but, instead, intervenes in a therapeutic way to treat the maladaptive response.

This treatment difference is based on the idea that depression following an injury, unlike grief, is a maladaptive response to the crisis of illness. As discussed in chapter 4, the distinction between grief and depression may be difficult to make, or there may be a mixture of the two processes.

The crisis of depression that may follow a burn or trauma has certain characteristics:

1. Psychic disequilibrium with confusion and uncertainty;
2. Regression with intensified transference;
3. A tendency to examine the trajectory of one's life—where one has been, where one is going, and which expectations will be fulfilled.

Viedermann and Perry contend that physically ill (or injured) patients are not only more vulnerable to depression but also more responsive to psychological intervention (11). They describe their intervention as a "psychodynamic life narrative" because it is a global statement about the meaning of the illness (injury) in the context of the patient's entire life, as opposed to the interpretation of a single conflict.

Although this technique was originally directed toward patients with physical illness, we have found it suitable for patients who have suffered a trauma or burn injury. As we have pointed out, pain control must first be achieved before any meaningful therapeutic interaction can be initiated.

Once pain is controlled, there needs to be an examination of the patient's present and past life, with emphasis on psychological factors and relationships. This can be done in two or three bedside consultation visits. Sometimes, especially since only abbreviated contact may be possible, several additional visits are required. During these contacts, the information gathered will ultimately be used in formulating the psychodynamic life narrative. This patient/therapist contact, taking place at a time when the patient is vulnerable and regressed, will also facilitate the natural transference that occurs under these circumstances. It is also likely that during these preliminary visits the therapist may be making suggestions concerning pain control, family matters, or other psychosocial issues.

At some point, the therapist will have enough information to make a psychodynamic life narrative interpretation to the patient. This statement explains what the injury means psychodynamically to the patient at a particular time. The degree of depression is usually viewed as a natural result of the patient's personal psychology rather than as an inevitable consequence of the injury per se.

This narrative statement is based on relatively limited contact with the patient and will thus be abbreviated and oversimplified. Viedermann and Perry believe that this simplification provides a cohesive structure (11). The psychic disorder produced by the crisis of injury can become organized around the coherent account of the patient's current personal experience and his or her plight in relation to the past.

The patient has a positive relationship with the therapist, founded in the regressed state that intensifies transference wishes. To gratify these wishes and reinforce positive past experience, the narrative should be presented in an engaging and vigorous manner that conveys fascination and interest in the patient, as well as affirmation and hope.

The narrative is designed to create a new perspective and to increase self-esteem through the emphasis of past strength, support, and coping mechanisms that have been effective. It can be used to point out that the depression is an understandable response when previous adaptive methods can no longer be used.

The narrative can help the patient accept where he or she is in the life cycle and understand the current state as something that had to be, as a realistic result of the accident or injury. The key to the approach is the presentation the therapist makes to the patient—the statement that places the injury in the context of the patient's life trajectory and demonstrates the psychodynamic logic of his depression.

CASE STUDY 2 (11)

A 17-year-old Chinese-American male high school student was hospitalized with 28% second- and third-degree burns over his face and upper body. The injury occurred while he was repairing his parents' basement furnace. The patient was not participating in physical therapy and was developing debilitating contractures. He was depressed and appeared to have given up and to have withdrawn into himself.

During a series of preliminary interviews exploring his background, the young man indicated that he did not think he deserved to recover. Ultimately, a psychodynamic life narrative was made that pointed out how he had always tried to be a good kid—plodding away at school, working part-time, and never arguing with anyone including his friends and family. He was told by the therapist it appeared he never got angry or lost his temper. "Of course, then, anger had to come out somewhere to keep you from exploding. It did come out in your dream that you had before the accident [a dream where the patient dreamed he had blown up his house]. Now, even though they found a defect in the welding equipment, you are convinced that your dream has come true and that you were trying to blow up your house. Because you have always been so good, you are now being extra hard on yourself for those angry feelings."

After the patient's suppressed anger had been placed in the context of his life and viewed as understandable adolescent rebelliousness, his depression began to lift and a therapeutic alliance was established for further work with the therapist.

CASE STUDY 3

A 31-year-old woman sustained multiple trauma in a motor vehicle accident. During the acute phase of treatment, she had to be in traction and on an electric bed that constantly rotates from side to side and had numerous I.V. lines running into her. She tolerated the sensory isolation unusually well but became depressed and tearful when she was moved into a regular bed and room. During preliminary interviews with the psychiatrist a history emerged. The patient was the youngest of several children and she felt neglected while growing up. She entertained herself by making up imaginary stories. Later on, in high school and college, she was told that she was a talented writer. After graduation, she chose to work in her father's lumberyard in an attempt to gain his approval. She had been thinking about going back to school to become a teacher or writer but could never bring herself to tell her father her wish. Her job required bookkeeping work, which she did not like, as well as considerable physical labor, which she would not be able to resume because of her injuries.

During the first part of hospitalization she tolerated the forced passivity by making up stories. She was surprised when the psychiatrist told her that her ability to sustain herself without breaking down during that initial period was highly unusual, and obviously due to her inner creativity. This made her more willing to reflect on becoming a writer.

In the psychodynamic narrative statement she was told, "You are now depressed because you believe that by not being able to work in the lumberyard you will disappoint your father and won't be a worthwhile person. Yet you know that you want to be a writer or a teacher and are better than most in these endeavors. The reality is that this injury means that you won't be able to be as physically active as before, but that you can do what you always wanted to do."

When the life narrative was elaborated on, the patient acknowledged that she felt neglected as a child. To make up for this situation, she suppressed her talents and her wish to be a writer or to teach others to write. She was trying to please her father by working in his business, which her brothers had refused to do.

The impact of this insight on the patient was quite dramatic. Her affect changed rapidly and she became quite receptive to the support of her family. She also began to reflect about the future in a more positive and realistic way.

Time-limited Psychotherapy

Experienced psychotherapists who work in the medical setting may wish to study the "time-limited psychotherapy" techniques of James Mann (12). This is a specific approach to short-term psychotherapy which, in the original description, utilizes 12 intense and focused therapy sessions. The method can be altered for the medical/surgical setting and can have therapeutic value in carefully selected situations. Trauma and burn patients who are medically stable often require continued hospitalizations for traction, rehabilitation, physiotherapy, occupational therapy, multiple grafting procedures, and so forth. These hospitalizations present an opportunity to do insight oriented short-term psychotherapeutic work with an appropriately chosen, well-motivated patient. We will briefly review this technique of psychotherapy as it applies to the burn and trauma patient.

An initial screening determines that the patient has a central conflict causing the anxiety depression, and that the conflict has often been reflected in interpersonal difficulties existing prior to the injury. Problems with authority figures, dependency relationships, and separation issues are common examples.

The presence of psychosis or profound depression is usually contraindicated in this technique. The patient should have a clear sensorium and be free of significant pain. Since this short-term psychotherapy approach usually involves a planned breaking off of contact with the psychotherapist at the conclusion of treatment, it might be advisable to have an alternate referral plan for patients expected to have long-term severe psychological repercussions due to the injury. This category of patients might include patients with major burns; significant injury to face, genitals, and breasts; and deforming injuries to arms and legs. In a similar manner, usually neither patients who are grieving a loved one lost in the accident, nor head trauma patients or patients with injury to the spinal cord who were seen during the initial injury phase would be considered for this technique.

Patients who have multiple fractures that require hospitalization for 6–12 weeks or patients who require numerous skin grafts meet the criteria for the time-limited treatment approach. Although we suggest that the central focus conflict should be one that predates the accident, it is expected that the accident, nature of injury, and events that occurred during hospitalization will be important parts of this psychotherapeutic work.

It is essential that the number of sessions planned and their duration be spelled out in advance. The usual technique, as described by Mann, is twelve 45-minute sessions, once a week. We have found it practical and workable to reduce the total number of sessions to six to eight and, sometimes, to reduce the time to 30 minutes per session. The exact time of each appointment, including the final date, should be clearly specified in advance. This is based on the idea that knowing the termination date at the start increases both the anxiety with respect to loss as well as the defenses against loss. The intensification of defenses against separation and loss serve to highlight much of the central conflict.

We suggest that the anticipated total number of sessions be kept constant. However, it may be practical to have sessions twice a week or to make up a particular session that may have been missed because of a test or procedure that had to be done. If discharge occurs prior to the termination date, there can be an agreement to complete the treatment as an outpatient, perhaps on the date when the follow-up visit to the hospital for medical/surgical care is scheduled.

The treatment technique is believed to be effective because the intense time limited treatment technique mobilizes transference. There is often rapid symptomatic improvement within the first three or four meetings. This "transference cure" should not be demeaned when it does take place and the treatment should be continued as planned. Then, the patient will try to avoid what he has avoided earlier in life—a "separation without resolution from the meaningful ambivalently experienced person." The fact that the patient is hospitalized enhances regression and brings out dependency conflicts.

Toward the end of therapy, the patient attempts to ward off separation, and the treatment deals with the patient's reaction to termination. Sadness, grief, anger, and guilt, with accompanying manifestations in fantasy and behavior, become the main focus of treatment. The patient is not only dealing with separation from a therapist and termination of therapy, but also separation from medical and surgical teams that provided given care when he or she was helpless and frightened. In fact, these persons may indeed have saved his or her life. Also included here is the separation from a myriad of specialists who have assisted recovery, as well as physical therapists and occupational therapists who have helped the patient to achieve recovery of function or adjust to new circumstances. An essential part of such psychotherapy is to examine feelings of termination as they relate to the present and the past. This will unavoidably become intertwined with the central conflict that had been the focus of the treatment.

The therapist involved in an intense time limited psychotherapy must deal with his or her own countertransference feelings. The therapist may also be going through a "separation without resolution." These feelings are of course related to the personal feelings of the therapist, but are also molded by the personality of the patient and the events of the hospitalization. An awareness of how a particular patient affects the therapist can be helpful in understanding how other medical staff respond to this patient. At discharge, the entire team goes through a separation. At times, the staff needs some help in dealing with its own reactions.

A CASE STUDY UTILIZING TIME-LIMITED THERAPY

A 28-year-old computer analyst severely injured both legs in a motorcycle accident. Three weeks after an elaborate attempt to save it, the right leg was amputated above the knee. During the initial period in the hospital, the patient concluded that his leg could not be saved and that his best chance for a speedy recovery and rehabilitation was amputation. He did grief work during this time and was thought to be as prepared as a person could be under the circumstances.

During the first postoperative week, he was optimistic about the future. He handled pain quite well and was making a good postoperative recovery. He became friendly with the house staff who were his age, but, by postoperative day 7, he was noted to be quite depressed. He was irritable and short-tempered. He was no longer cooperative with the nurses and only half-heartedly participated in bedside physical therapy. He acknowledged that he felt depressed, but could not verbalize any particular ideation. His appetite was satisfactory and there were no significant sleep problems.

At this point, a psychiatric consultation was held with a member of the consultation liaison group who had not seen the patient previously. After initial discussion, the patient and the therapist agreed to meet for a half-hour therapy session twice a week for the next 4 weeks, for a total of eight half-hour meetings. It was anticipated that the patient would remain in the hospital during this time for skin grafting on his left leg and for the beginning of rehabilitation for his right let. It was also understood that the therapy would be short and intensive. The goal was to clarify and to alleviate his feelings of depression and to help him cope with his current situation. The patient was not interested in long-term follow-up, and understood that the current therapist would not be available after the planned sessions were completed.

Sessions 1–2. There was an elaboration and open-ended exploration of the patient's background. He was the youngest of three sons. His father was a high-powered attorney and his mother was a nurse who was very dedicated to volunteering for charity work and helping disadvantaged persons. He grew up in a warm household, but the atmosphere was competitive, with high expectations. His older brothers went directly to law school after college. He took 6 years to finish college, spending 2 years in Colorado trying "to find myself and help people." After graduation, he preferred to work alone and set up a computer consulting business that proved to be quite helpful to small firms and stores, and which gave him considerable pleasure. He had numerous girl friends, but said that he didn't want to settle down until he was "successful." He talked about the loss of his leg, and his grief work seemed appropriate and free flowing.

Sessions 3–4. The patient was relating well. He enjoyed talking with his therapist, especially about a software program he was writing with his computer at the bedside. He contemplated designing medically oriented programs. He was, however, still quite pessimistic about his future. He did not talk about the rehabilitation activity and seemed uninterested in plans that were being worked out for him.

A life narrative interpretation was made to the patient. In the interpretation, it was pointed out that the patient desired to help people, as his mother did, and received satisfaction when he could be helpful. In the hospital he had suffered a major loss and required people to help him. Both of these factors made him feel less of a person and diminished his self-esteem. He responded to the interpretation with interest and spoke a great deal about these points. While he became more cooperative and seemed to receive assistance more easily, he was still depressed and unable to verbalize what was disturbing him.

Sessions 5–6. He appeared to look forward to visits with the therapist. He related a dream that suggested a wish to walk again, and enjoyed discussions with the therapist about the meaning of the dream. He was participating in some of the planning of his outpatient rehabilitation program. However, he did make unfriendly, hostile remarks to some of the housestaff with whom he had been close during the earlier part of his hospitalization. At the end of session

6, when the therapist reminded him they would only have two more sessions together, the patient suggested that they should terminate immediately after that session. The therapist emphatically told him that it was not a good idea and proposed that it would be useful to spend the next two sessions talking about his response to the staff, which included the therapist. The therapist also suggested that such discussions would help the patient understand how he was dealing with his amputation and rehabilitation plans. The patient was surprised at the therapist's suggestion, but agreed.

Sessions 7–8. The housestaff had rotated since the last session and the patient noted how these staff members had all gone on to "bigger and better things." He could relate this to his own family life—everyone was expected to go to college and beyond. The patient shared his feelings: He was angry that the therapist would not be able to see him through his rehabilitation.

The anticipated termination of the psychotherapy with the expected separation from the therapist and hospital staff was meaningful to him. He felt he did not have an opportunity to show these persons that he was going to have a good recovery. He also regretted that he could not complete his software program for the hospital staff. These feelings, following the loss of his leg, were a big blow to his self-esteem.

With the help of the therapist, he was able to understand that he was repeating his earlier disappointments in life when he could not match his brothers' accomplishments or please his parents by being high-powered enough for his father and "helping" enough for his mother. By accepting this insight, he was now able to see that he had actually achieved the admiration and respect of many of the doctors and nurses who had cared for him, as he had always earned the admiration of persons who knew him well.

His anger at the therapist was diminished when he was reminded that the purpose of eight sessions was to give him insight into his coping ability, which it did. He felt very good about what he had accomplished in this time.

The eight-session time-limited therapy allowed the patient to have an intense emotional experience at a time when he was vulnerable to regressed feelings. This method allowed him to uncover an understanding of some of his depressive reactive symptoms. The anticipation of the termination of this therapy and the sensitive handling of his reactions to this experience gave him personal insight that would be helpful as he continued to cope with his injury.

ALL HOSPITAL PSYCHOTHERAPY AS TIME LIMITED

The applicability of Mann's formal techniques involves the identification of a pre-existing central psychological conflict and requires a focused insight-oriented therapy. This is not the treatment of choice for most patients hospitalized with burn and trauma. Rather than focus on underlying psychological conflicts, most psychotherapeutic work with burn and trauma patients deals with the patient's psychological reactions to injury and to the hospitalization. Nevertheless, the nature of Mann's time-limited psychotherapy, described previously, has important applicability to many patients.

For some patients, the promise of regular follow-up visits by the psychotherapist fosters a diminution of many psychological symptoms. The role of the psychotherapist may be primarily supportive, showing empathy and facilitating abreaction, or it may be mixed. The mental health professional is an advocate for better pain control, a facilitator of improved family communication, and a provider of some psychotherapy.

The anticipated discharge date in most cases brings up powerful feelings on the part of the patient. The patient anticipates discharge with great joy and happiness and as a major step toward recovery. However, discharge stirs up the patient's insecurities about his ability to function outside of the hospital and without the caregivers. The patient is concerned about others' responses to his appearance or any altered body function. Then there are the inevitable personal attachments to individual staff members, based on real relationships that formed during this critical period and based on transference relationships facilitated by the regressed dependency position of the hospitalized patient. Separation anxiety and certain degrees of sadness are present in anticipation of discharge. It is often quite helpful if the therapeutic work includes an insight-oriented approach about these issues.

For other patients, just recognizing feelings of separation can be a support. Patients can be reassured that their feelings are normal and likely to resolve, and that there is an open invitation to visit the therapist after discharge. This opportunity to make a follow-up appointment is supportive to some patients.

Referral for Additional Therapy

Often, psychotherapeutic contact in the hospital is quite limited. Problems of pain control and transient organic brain syndrome are treated symptomatically. Some brief psychotherapeutic work may focus on adjustment to the burn or injury. Often, patients who previously had never considered talking to a mental health professional find themselves confiding inner thoughts and emotions to them during hospitalization. The interaction with the mental health professional provides an example of what it would be like to do further psychotherapy work after discharge from the hospital. The contact in the hospital is also an opportunity to help the patient identify psychological problems that deserve follow-up care. Symptoms of anxiety, depression, and panic, and substance abuse and marital problems are common issues that can be recognized during the hospitalization and that require further treatment.

Frequently, the mental health professional's contact with the patient is geared toward helping the patient deal with resistance to needed psychotherapy. On occasion, there may be a question of whether a patient is suicidal or needs immediate psychiatric hospitalization because of dangerous behavior or an inability to function due to psychological problems. In such situations, a psychiatrist should be brought in immediately or certainly before discharge if one has not been already involved in the consultation.

For most patients, any referral will be for outpatient treatment. If the consultant does outpatient therapy, then it would be ideal for him or her to continue treatment with the patient. There are exceptions to this approach. Occasionally, a particular patient may displace onto the therapist negative feelings that have not been recognized or adequately interpreted. In this situation, a different mental health professional should follow-up with the patient. Also, in the case of Mann's time-limited therapy described above, the therapist has set an enforced termination as part of the treatment technique and would not be encouraging the patient to return for follow-up. As previously mentioned, even with this approach, when psychological sequelae are expected, a referral to another therapist could be made.

In addition, if the inpatient consultant is not available for outpatient treatment because of time constraints, geography, financial considerations, or for other reasons, the referral will ultimately be made to another person or clinic. By building on the relationship made in the hospital with the consultant or psychosocial team, the referral will be more effective.

It is not unusual for a patient to agree to a follow-up appointment and not keep it, or to accept a referral and not call for an appointment. Frequently, the patient cannot anticipate how he or she will feel on returning to the home environment after hospitalization. Not only will the patient's attention be more divided, but the psychological equilibrium and motivation for psychological follow-up will change.

To avoid making an appointment with the patient that will not be kept, or to avoid spending time discussing a referral with an outside colleague who will never be called by the patient, the following technique is suggested. Give the patient the phone number of the consultant or of a member of the psychosocial team with whom he or she has established a working reliance during hospitalization. Encourage the patient to *call* for a follow-up appointment or for a referral, preferably within 1–2 weeks after arriving home. (Patients can also be encouraged to call and report how they are doing even if they are not going to request a follow-up appointment.)

Despite patients' best intentions at the time of discharge, and good working relationships during hospitalization notwithstanding, in our experience, less than one-quarter of the patients who agree to do so will actually call for an appointment or referral. Most patients are pleased to receive this offer, and they tell us that even carrying our phone number is comforting and supportive. However, if the patient calls for an appointment, he or she is likely to keep it. If a patient does ask for a referral after discharge, it can be assumed that he or she is highly motivated and will follow up. Under these circumstances, after receiving the patient's call, we make immediate efforts to give the patient a definite appointment. If we are going to refer the patient to a colleague or clinic, an advance telephone call to our colleague is made to pave the way once we receive the patient's call. We inform our colleague of the motivation the patient has demonstrated by calling us for a referral.

Death and Dying

How best to help the patient who reaches the point of inevitable death following a major burn or trauma is always a difficult question. While the topic has been considered briefly in Chapter 3, on emergency room interventions, the subject deserves further discussion. Today, a multitude of books exist on the subject of death and dying, yet a gap remains in the training and sense of competence of medical personnel who face issues of loss or threatened loss of life. Even the most highly trained member of the mental health team may not feel comfortable coping with death or supporting those experiencing the end of life.

Perhaps the most common fears of the dying person are the fear of being in pain and of being alone. Pain, while not easy to address, can be managed through techniques discussed in Chapter 1. The fear of being alone is less easily remedied. First, one must clarify exactly what is meant by the patient's fear of being alone. "Don't let me be alone" could mean that the patient wants the family or medical personnel at the bedside or that he or she simply does not want to be isolated and abandoned as many patients are when professionals are no longer able to define their roles.

Elizabeth Kubler-Ross, who has written extensively about the experience of dying persons, reports that she feels fully comfortable telling her patients that they will not be alone, based on her extensive experience with sudden death (3). Patients who have had a sudden death experience (and then were revived) consistently reported to her not a feeling of aloneness, but an experience of either being with others whom they have known and who have preceded them in death, or a vague sort of joining with some "presence." We do not advocate any one particular approach or set of words that is most helpful, but rather a continued attendance of the patient. Even when the patient seems unaware and unable to respond to support, the staff can speak comforting words. The most important role of the mental health professional may be to notice the isolation of the patient or the premature withdrawal of the patient's support. While staff members may report a sense of helplessness about what they can offer the patient, they may need to be reminded of their role in helping the family with its expression of anticipatory grief and acceptance of the approaching end of life. The staff can begin to help the family with concrete plans and the recourse to already established support systems.

References

1. Stedeford A. Facing death—patients, families, and professionals. Oxford: Heinemann Medical Books, 1984, p. 154.
2. Kubler-Ross E. On death and dying. New York: Macmillan, 1969.
3. Kubler-Ross E. Questions on death and dying. New York: Macmillan, 1974.
4. Kubler-Ross E. Death: the final stage of growth. New York: Macmillan, 1975.
5. Westberg GE. Good grief—a constructive approach to the problem of loss. Philadelphia: Fortress Press, 1962.
6. Lindemann E. Symptomatology and management of acute grief. Am J Psychiatry 1944; 101:141–148.
7. Davidson GW. Understanding mourning—a guide to those who grieve. Minneapolis: Augsberg Publishing House, 1984.
8. Tempereau C, Grossman RA, Brones M. Psychological regression and marital status: determinants in psychiatric management of burn victims. J. Burn Care Rehabil 1987;8:286–291.
9. Carnes B. Concept analysis: dependence. Crit Care Q 1984;29–39.
10. Blumenfield M. Patients' fantasies about physical illness. Psychother Psychosom 1983; 39:171–179.
11. Viedermann M, Perry SW. Use of psychodynamic life narrative in the treatment of depression in the physically ill. Gen Hosp Psychiatr 1980;3:177–185.
12. Mann J. Time-limited psychotherapy. Cambridge, MA: Harvard University Press, 1973.

6

Use of Psychotropic Drugs

Psychotropic medications and their use are mentioned in various chapters in this book. This chapter discusses some general principles and reviews some specific characteristics of various medications. It is *not* meant to be a complete primer of psychopharmacology. It is important that the treating physician become familiar with all indications, contraindications, adverse reactions, drug interactions, and dosage schedules of any medication being prescribed. This can be done by referring to the PDR, manufacturer's updates, and inserts that provide more complete information. The nursing staff must also be well acquainted with the characteristics of drugs being used in its unit and this knowledge of drugs should be updated regularly.

Antidepressants

Acute burn and trauma injuries are often life-threatening. Under these circumstances, the administration, immediate readministration, or maintenance of antidepressant drugs is of secondary importance for the patient's welfare. Of prime concern is the stabilization of the patient's medical condition and the provision of adequate pain control. Frequently, such a patient has suffered a severe assault to the cardiovascular and central nervous system, with major metabolic impact. The patient's condition will be further complicated by new drugs, blood, and other fluid infusions, and, possibly, by anesthetization and surgical intervention. The patient may have an altered state of consciousness and be in physical and emotional shock. The concern and empathy for the patient's emotional plight at this time should not precipitate premature use of psychotropic medication.

There is little value in using antidepressant medication in the early phase of an injury. Side effects of the drugs can complicate the stability of the critically ill patient. Many of these drugs have a tendency to sedate, which would be synergistic with pain medication and could possibly lead to the underutilization of pain medication at a time when every effort should be made to achieve definitive pain control.

When the patient's medical condition and pain are stabilized, it may be appropriate to consider the role of various psychotropic medications in the treatment plan. Side effects, onset of action, and drug interactions, as well as the potential benefit of medication at this point, need to be carefully considered. When properly used, antidepressive medication can be effective in alleviating the symptoms of depressive illness, including sadness and hopelessness. These drugs may also diminish feelings of worthlessness and guilt. As the depressive symptoms subside, the patient may experience an improvement in energy level as well as a decrease in fatigue and the disappearance of suicidal thoughts.

Decisions concerning when and how to use antidepressant medication must be made by the burn or trauma team and the psychiatric consultant. It is also necessary to evaluate patients in a burn or trauma unit who at the time of injury are already on psychotropic drugs.

DANGERS OF MONOAMINE OXIDASE INHIBITORS

If it is determined that an acute trauma or burn patient has a psychiatric history or was on antidepressive medication at the time of the accident, there should be an immediate determination of whether the patient was taking monoamine oxidase inhibitors (MAOIs) such as tranylcypromine (Parnate), isocarboxazid (Marplan), phenelzine (Nardil), and others. This is essential. A patient who receives meperidine (Demerol) for pain control and who is also on MAOIs or had been on them even 2 or 3 weeks previously can have serious reactions such as coma, severe hypertension or hypotension, severe respiratory depression, convulsions, malignant hyperexia, peripheral vascular collapse, and death. These reactions may be mediated by the accumulation of 5-HT (serotonin) consequent to MAOIs (1, 2).

General anesthesia can be a problem as can local anesthesia containing sympathomimetic vasoconstrictors. Patients on MAOIs are also particularly vulnerable to the effects of sympathomimetics that inhibit certain enzymes. These sympathomimetics include compounds such as levodopa, dopamine, reserpine, methyldopa, and others. These drugs and several others may cause a hypertensive crisis in a patient on MAOIs. If a hypertensive crisis occurs, immediate medical consultation should be obtained. On the basis of present evidence, the slow administration of phentolamine (Regitine), 5 mg I.V., is the treatment of choice for this condition (1). No interaction is expected with direct-acting sympathomimetics such as epinephrine, isoproterenol, norepinephrine, or methoxamine.

There should be at least 2 weeks between discontinuation of most other antidepressants and administration of an MAOI and there should be a 5-week interval between an MAOI and fluoxetine (Prozac).

Other important drug interactions and diet considerations must be considered with any patient on an MAOI. MAOIs can be excellent antidepressants, but, because of the issue raised above, they are rarely used in treatment with burn and trauma patients, except as a secondary choice when no adverse interaction is expected.

TRICYCLIC ANTIDEPRESSANTS

The history and current use of any antidepressant medication in an acute burn or trauma patient should alert the treatment team to the possibility of the patient's depressive response to the injury. This history and use, however, do *not* constitute a call for the immediate continuation or reinstitution of this medication. It takes 2–5 weeks for the body to eliminate an existing antidepressant. Even under nontraumatic situations, the cessation of such a medication does not necessarily bring about an immediate return of severe depressive symptoms. When deciding to reinstitute antidepressive medication, the possible early return of depressive symptoms must be weighed against drug interactions and potential adverse effects, such as postural hypotension, sedation, anticholinergic effects, and others described below.

Will the patient be undergoing immediate surgical procedures under anesthesia? If so, most anesthesiologists prefer that the patient be off antidepressants for at least 2 weeks before surgery to avoid drug interactions. If the acute trauma or burn patient presents severe depressive symptoms, the close observation standard in an intensive care setting or in one-to-one nursing care can adequately address the concern for a potentially suicidal patient until appropriate drug and psychotherapy measures can be instituted.

We have discussed elsewhere some of the difficulties in assessing depression in acutely injured burn or medically ill patients. Antidepressive medication should not replace needed supportive psychotherapeutic intervention. However, even when there is no presenting underlying major affective disorder, it may be determined that a trial of antidepressive medication is beneficial to a patient with severe, persistent depressive symptoms. This medication is usually instituted when the medical condition has stabilized and pain control has been adequately achieved.

In choosing antidepressants, the treating physician must consider the side effect profile and contraindications of each medication (see Table 6.1).

Table 6.1. Antidepressive Drugs[a]

Drugs—Class	Therapeutic Dose Range mg/day	Anticholinergic Effects	Sedation Effects
Tricyclics—tertiary amines			
Amitriptyline (Elavil)	50–300	+ + + + +	+ + + + +
Imipramine (Toframil)	50–300	+ + + +	+ + +
Triimpramine (Surmontil)	50–300	+ + + +	+ + + +
Doxepin (Sinequan)	50–300	+ + +	+ + + +
Tricyclics—secondary amines			
Nortriptyline (Aventyl, Pamelor)	25–200	+ +	+ +
Desipramine (Norpramin)	50–300	+	+
Protriptyline (Vivactil, Triptil)	30–60	+ + +	+ +
Tricyclic dibenzoxazepine			
Amoxapine (Asendin)	100–400	+ +	+ +
Tetracyclic			
Maprotiline (Ludiomil)	75–225	+	+ + + +
Triazolopyridine			
Trazodone (Desyrel)	100–400	+	+ + + + +
Monocyclic			
Bupropion (Wellbutrin)	225–400		+
Bicyclic			
Fluoxetine (Prozac)	20–60	+	+

[a] This chart is based on a composite of various published studies and charts (11, 14), and our own clinical experience.

CARDIOVASCULAR CONSIDERATIONS

The tricyclic antidepressants are known to prolong conduction time and thus prolong PR and QRS intervals on the electrocardiogram at or just above therapeutic plasma levels. In patients free of bundle branch disease, these changes in the electrocardiogram are rarely if ever clinically significant at normal therapeutic plasma levels of antidepressant. Patients who have presenting bundle branch block are at risk for developing second- or third-degree block, and need to be closely monitored if tricyclic antidepressants are initiated (3).

Tricyclic antidepressants have quinidine-like effects, and thus have the type I antiarrhythmic properties that inhibit fast sodium channels and, therefore, prolong the refractory period of the action potential of the cardiac conduction system. This effect tends to suppress ectopic pacemakers that are thought to cause atrial flutter, atrial fibrillation, ventricular tachycardia, and premature ventricular contractions (4, 5). These consequences can add to the effect of the other antiarrhythmics the patient may be receiving. Trazodone has been associated with arrhythmia in patients with pre-existing cardiac disease.

Tricyclic antidepressants can induce postural hypotension, an important problem in the elderly and in patients with pre-existing cardiovascular disease. The drugs of this class that are less likely to create this effect are the secondary amines—desipramine (Norpramin), the metabolite of imipramine (Tofranil); and nortriptyline (Pamelor), the metabolite of amitriptyline (Elavil). When there is cardiovascular disease, the selective serotonin reuptake inhibitors, such as fluoxetine (Prozac) and sertraline (Zoloft) may be an appropriate choice as an antidepressive medication.

ANTICHOLINERGIC EFFECTS

Anticholinergic side effects are among the most important adverse aspects of tricyclic antidepressants. Patients on tricyclics may also be receiving other drugs, such as antiparkinsonian agents, antihistamines, and neuroleptics, with anticholinergic effects. This combination may increase the risk of hypothermia, delirium, or both.

Constipation of varying degrees is a common anticholinergic side effect of most of the tricyclic antidepressants. Constipation, a major side effect of morphine and other narcotic analgesics that a patient may receive, is also exacerbated by diet and lack of exercise in the bedridden patient. This side effect usually can easily be treated by increasing bulk and fluid intake, and by administering stool softeners and laxatives. Referral to the protocol for bowel regimens in the chapter on pain and its management may be helpful.

Although less common than constipation, urinary retention and delayed micturition may occur in uncatheterized patients receiving tricyclic antidepressants. Management with bethanechol can be considered. Close attention to the overall medical condition, renal function, use of diuretics, and fluid management are, of course, important in the management of any burn and trauma patient.

Narrow-angle glaucoma may be exacerbated by antidepressants with anticholinergic side effects. However, patients with open angle glaucoma are at minimal risk. Even patients with narrow angle glaucoma can take tricyclics if ophthalmological consultants monitor intraocular pressure. Antidepressants without anticholinergic properties such as fluoxetine (Prozac) and sertraline (Zoloft) may be preferable in this situation.

SEIZURE POTENTIAL

Maprotiline (Ludomil), a tetracyclic antidepressant, is known to produce seizures in nonepileptic patients with doses above 200 mg/day and with rapid loading doses (4). All the tricyclics may have a tendency to lower seizure thresholds. Among the tricyclic agents, amitriptyline (Elavil) appears more likely to aggravate seizures (6). Bupropion (Wellbutrin) carries a greater risk of seizures than other antidepressants and is generally avoided in patients with epilepsy and in other high-risk patients—for example, those with a history of head trauma or with foci on the electroencephalogram (EEG) indicating potentially enhanced central nervous system irritability (4, 7). In fact, any patient with a history of head trauma or known brain damage should receive an EEG prior to antidepressant therapy. Those with significant paroxysmal EEG abnormalities should receive prophylactic anticonvulsants.

SEDATION AND AGITATION

The tertiary amines, mainly amitriptyline, imipramine, trimipramine, and doxepin, are the most sedative of the tricyclic antidepressants. Trazodone (Desyrel) and maprotiline are also quite sedative, as are MAOIs. This effect is especially important to consider when a patient receives other sedating medication including narcotics, benzodiazepines, neuroleptics, hypnotics, antihistamines, and barbiturates. If sedation is a problematic side effect, it may be possible to give most or all dosage in the evening. With paradoxical agitation, a less common side effect, it may be possible to give the dosage early in the day. Fluoxetine (Prozac) more likely produces agitation or insomnia and is usually given in the early morning.

PRIAPISM

Trazodone has been associated with the rare occurrence of priapism. In approximately one-third of the reported cases of this adverse effect, surgical intervention was required. In a portion of these cases, permanent impairment of erectile function or impotence resulted.

DRUG INTERACTIONS

Several important potential drug interactions have already been discussed. There should always be careful consideration of drug interactions when a patient is on multiple drugs. The description in this section is not meant to be comprehensive. Refer to the PDR or other sources whenever new drugs are added to a patient treatment plan.

Yet unmentioned is the possible decrease of antihypertensive effect in a patient who also receives cyclic antidepressants and antihypertensive medication, such as reserpine, guanethidine, and others. Hypotension can be augmented in patients on thiazide diuretics and acetazolamide. Hypertensives such as epinephrine, norepinephrine, and phenylephrine can cause enhanced pressor response. Patients receiving warfarin may have increased bleeding when they receive cyclic antidepressants. Increased serum digoxin or phenytoin levels have been reported in patients receiving trazodone with warfarin or tricyclic antidepressants.

Because fluoxetine is tightly bound to plasma protein, its administration to a patient taking another drug that is tightly bound to protein (i.e., warfarin, digitoxin, or others) may cause a shift in plasma concentrations, with a potentially adverse effect. Conversely, adverse effects may result from the displacement of protein bound fluoxetine by other tightly bound drugs. Patients receiving fluoxetine and lithium may have altered lithium levels.

The potentially dangerous interaction between MAOIs and narcotics, especially meperidine, has already been described. It is also important not to administer cyclic antidepressants with an MAOI, which should be discontinued for at least 10–14 days before starting the antidepressant. There should be a discontinuation of fluoxetine for 5 weeks before instituting an MAOI, and there should be a respite of at least a week between the administration of various MAOIs. The use of the muscle relaxant succinylcholine while an MAOI is in the body may prolong apnea (4). As previously mentioned, it would be highly unlikely to institute an MAOI in the acute trauma and burn patient, but patients may enter the hospital already on them.

Thyroid medication may potentiate any antidepressant effect, although it is not clear if this effect is due to an alleviation of the depression that is secondary to subclinical hypothyroidism.

LIVER DISEASE

Primary liver disease and secondary liver involvement with other diseases, such as congestive heart failure, may result in a less rapid metabolism of cyclic antidepressants and thus a longer half-life than is seen in a normally healthy population. A number of drugs, including cimetidine, which is frequently given to trauma and burn patients, may inhibit hepatic enzymes and, thereby, increase the plasma level of cyclic antidepressants (4).

TREATMENT TECHNIQUE

The onset of action of antidepressant effect for these medications is usually 2–3 weeks, with an occasional patient requiring several weeks before therapeutic effect is achieved. Amoxapine appears to show antidepressant effects within the first week. Many side effects can have rapid onset. Changes in sleep patterns frequently occur within the first few days. When there is improvement of sleep, patients often report feeling less depressed. As noted in the chapter on pain, there are reports of tricyclic antidepressants having analgesic effects with fairly rapid onset.

In the physically debilitated patient, it is common to start with a low dosage and to titrate gradually, with careful attention to side effects and adverse reactions. Therefore, achievement of therapeutic effect may take longer in burn and trauma patients.

With one or two exceptions, it appears that blood levels correlate linearly with the therapeutic effect. The usual technique, then, would be to gradually increase dosage (within the usual range for that drug) until a therapeutic effect is achieved or until there are unacceptable side effects. Nortriptyline is an exception. Its therapeutic antidepressant effect falls within a window of between 50 and 150 mg/ml for the blood level. Amitriptyline breaks down to nortriptyline, thus both the primary drug and the metabolite are present in the bloodstream. It is questionable whether a similar window exists for the combined value of both substances.

Geriatric patients often require lower dosages. There may be some analgesic or antipruritic effects at lower dosages. Doxepin, trimipramine, and amitriptyline have strong antihistaminic effects and so may be helpful in patients with severe itching.

Occasionally, when measuring nortriptyline and desipramine levels in burn patients, we have noted unexpectedly low or very high levels. We expect that this may be due to an unusual alteration of the metabolism of the burn patient.

We have found that the secondary amines, nortriptyline and desipramine, are usually the best tolerated of the tricyclics. We have recently gained experience with fluoxetine and find that this drug may have many advantages in the medical setting because of its low side-effect profile. Its characteristic of affecting the blood level of other drugs (as previously discussed) must be taken into account.

Benzodiazepines

The benzodiazepines have important uses during all phases of the treatment of the burn and trauma patient. Anxiety is encountered at every turn, with potential for the utilization of this class of medication for its excellent anxiolytic qualities.

The benzodiazepines have a synergistic sedative effect with most analgesic medications, particularly the narcotic group, which is commonly used in the treatment of the trauma and burn patient. Because narcotics and benzodiazepines have an additive effect, there must be caution concerning oversedation or respiratory depression. Anxiety accompanies most painful states and also lowers the pain threshold. Therefore, clinicians frequently use benzodiazepines in combination with analgesics with appropriate caution. However, by themselves, the benzodiazepines are not true analgesics and should not be used as substitutes for adequate pain control. Tolerance to the sedative effect of the benzodiazepines does develop. The drowsiness that many patients report diminishes after a few days, despite the increasing plasma level concentrations of the benzodiazepines. There does not appear to be any clear tolerance to the antianxiety effect.

The decision to use benzodiazepines, and which one of them to use, must always take into account the patient's overall medical condition and current physical symptoms. Symptoms such as dizziness, difficulty breathing, rapid heartbeat, and so forth may actually reflect an existing medical condition, not anxiety. In such a situation, the underlying medical condition must be addressed first, and care should be taken not to mask conditions such as impending shock, sepsis, abnormal metabolic and endocrine states, and so forth. Nevertheless, even in the presence of medical illness, burn, or trauma, there may be a role for the careful use of tranquilizers, including benzodiazepines, as long as they are not employed to suppress symptoms that could be better treated by other medical means.

As described in the chapter, "Organic Mental Syndrome," the control of agitation in the delirious patient may be accomplished by the use of benzodiazepines, neuroleptics, or, sometimes, by the two combined. However, one of the reasons for extreme caution is that the underlying toxic state or medical condition, or other drugs being taken, may cause sedation to occur in unpredictable cycles. As discussed with narcotics, such combinations could produce an unwanted effect of oversedation. Aspiration is particularly dangerous in an oversedated patient.

It is also possible that a patient may already have been suffering from an anxiety disorder, possibly a panic disorder, before the trauma or burn injury. More recently, alprazolam has been approved by the Food and Drug Administration as an effective method of treating panic disorder and an increasing number of patients are being put on this drug for treatment of this condition. An estimated 0.5 to 1.0% of the population have some type of anxiety disorder (8). These conditions can be exacerbated by a trauma or burn injury and by some of the concomitant reactive psychodynamic factors mentioned in the chapter, "Psychological Reactions." When feasible in the medical setting, benzodiazepines may be the treatment of choice for these patients.

In some instances, a patient with an anxiety disorder who is on therapeutic doses of benzodiazepines may sustain a burn or trauma injury and suddenly be hospitalized, either in a conscious or unconscious state. It is then necessary to decide whether to continue such medication or to be prepared for possible benzodiazepine withdrawal if these anxiolytics are discontinued.

In addition to the treatment of anxiety, benzodiazepines are used to treat sleep disturbances. This symptom complex is seen in the trauma and burn patient as well as in patients who have anxiety and depressive symptoms. Certain benzodiazepines are designated as hypnotics because of particular characteristics, but, in reality, all drugs in this group can be used to promote sleep.

Frequently, benzodiazepines are used in a single administration for procedures such as endoscopy, bronchoscopy, dressing and cast changes, and so forth. The purpose is to relieve anxiety, enhance analgesia, and achieve short-term sedation. While any of the benzodiazepines could be used for this purpose, diazepam, lorazepam, alprazolam, and oxazepam are the most commonly used. If the procedure is expected to be painful, an analgesic is also given.

In regard to painful procedures, special mention should be made of the occasional use of Versed (midazolam), a high-potency benzodiazepine with a half-life of less than 3 hours (9). Versed I.M. or I.V. is used to achieve sedation in less than 15 minutes. The patient usually has a fairly complete anterograde amnesia. Versed is sometimes employed in burn and trauma patients as a preanesthetic or is used to produce amnesia for unpleasant or painful procedures such as endoscopy or dressing changes. This is not a common choice, because respiratory arrest is a concern and an anesthesiologist's presence is required during drug administration. When Versed is used and adequate analgesia is not given, the patient may scream, but will usually have no conscious memory of the procedure after it is over. We question, however, whether the overall experience may nevertheless register in some way in the unconscious and possibly have some adverse psychological effects. We suggest that adequate analgesia be the goal of treatment with any painful procedures.

Benzodiazepines have other functions that are appropriate in the burn and trauma patient. They have antiseizure qualities and can be used along with anticonvulsive medications for this purpose. Benzodiazepines have muscle-relaxing qualities and can be used for relieving muscle spasm as well as for the adjunctive treatment of extra pyramidal reactions to neuroleptic medication.

Benzodiazepines are also the treatment of choice for alcohol withdrawal syndromes, as discussed later in the chapter on alcohol and other substance abuse.

CHOICE OF A SPECIFIC BENZODIAZEPINE

There are few differences in the clinical efficacies of the various benzodiazepines. The side effects are quite similar and the choice of the drug is usually made on the basis of pharmacokinetics, although there are many variations in the expected parameters in different people. While there appear to be situations that favor short- versus long-acting drugs, serum levels of drugs metabolized by oxidation can be adjusted by using lower doses or decreased frequency of dosing (4) (see Table 6.2).

Short-acting agents such as alprazolam, lorazepam, or oxazepam are generally used for acute anxiety, especially for that which occurs during the performance of a frightening or painful procedure, as described above. However, this is not always the case: I.V. Valium, which has a long half-life, has a long history of use to control agitation and acute situational anxiety. Alprazolam appears to have a slightly more rapid onset of activity compared to oxazepam and lorazepam (10).

Long-acting agents such as chlordiazepoxide, diazepam, chlorazepate, prazepam, and clonazepam are initially considered in chronic anxiety conditions that require continuous drug effects. However, exceptions can easily be found. For example, as previously stated, alprazolam given three or four times a day regularly has been demonstrated to be effective for treating chronic panic disorders.

The benzodiazepines tend to be highly soluble and persist longer in obese individuals or in those individuals, such as the elderly, whose fat-to-lean body mass ratio is increased (11).

As a general rule, in the medically ill patient with complications and when drug interactions are likely, it is usually safer to have on board a short-acting substance that can be eliminated from the system quickly and whose levels can be easily controlled. Similarly, with debilitated burn and trauma patients who require benzodiazepine, it is better to give the smallest

Table 6.2. Commonly Used Benzodiazepines[a]

Name	Daily Range (mg)	Equivalent Dose of 1 mg Lorazepam	Elimination Half-life (Includes Active Metabolites When Taken P.O.) (h)	Peak Plasma Level When Taken P.O. (h)	Potency	Primary Metabolic Pathway
Short-acting						
Alprazolam (Xanax)	0.25–5.0	0.50	6–20	1–2	High	Oxidation
Lorazepam (Ativan)	0.50–6.0	1.00	8–25	2–3	High	Conjugation
Oxazepam (Serax)	10.0–60.0	15.00	5–21	2–3	Low	Conjugation
Tempazepam (Restoril)	15.0–30.0	10.00	9.5–24	2–3	Low	Conjugation
Triazolam (Halcion)	0.125–0.5	0.25	2–4.5	1–2	High	Oxidation
Long-acting						
Chlordiazepoxide (Librium)	5.0–100.00	25.00	28–120	1.0–4.0	Low	Conjugation
Clonazepam (Klonopin)	0.5–5.0	0.25	18–60	1.0–4.0	High	Conjugation
Chlorazepate (Tranxene)	7.5–60.0	10.00	50–120	1.0–4.0	Low	Oxidation
Diazepam (Valium)	2.0–60.0	5.00	28–150	1.0–2.0	Low	Oxidation
Flurazepam (Dalmane)	15.0–30.0	15.00	24–120	2.0–4.0	Low	Oxidation
Prazepam (Centrax)	20.0–60.0	10.00	24–200	2.5–6.0	Low	Oxidation

[a] This table is based on a composite of various published studies and tables (4, 9, 10, 16, 19) and our own clinical experience.

possible dose and to repeat that dose frequently if needed. The dosage can then be titrated upward to achieve the desired therapeutic effect.

BENZODIAZEPINES FOR SLEEP

Benzodiazepines shorten sleep latency and increase sleep continuity and are, therefore, good hypnotics. Short-acting benzodiazepines, such as triazolam and temazepam, are generally the hypnotics of choice. The former may have a slightly more rapid onset; the latter peaks slightly later. Some patients are more responsive to one than to another. Flurazepam has been used as an effective hypnotic. Its pharmacokinetic profile may be appropriate for late awakenings. However, as noted previously, the longer the half-life of a benzodiazepine, the greater the likelihood of a "hangover sedation" during the day.

Hypnotics are usually prescribed on a p.r.n. basis, although they may be given daily for several days when it is desirable to break an insomnia pattern. Care must be taken not to continually write a p.r.n. sleep order that is being used every night and may be carried over on a chronic basis. It is easier to prevent this from happening if the patient is informed, at an early date, that it is not necessary to take hypnotics on a daily basis and that hypnotics are usually more effective on a sporadic p.r.n. schedule. When necessary, if the benzodiazepine schedule is being reduced, patients should be reminded that, although they may be restless for a night or two and may actually have difficulty sleeping, this does not place their health in jeopardy and may be a necessary step toward a drug-free sleep pattern.

As expected, benzodiazepines as a group reduce the number of awakenings. The time in rapid eye movement (REM) sleep tends to be diminished, but the number of cycles of REM usually increases. With regular use of a benzodiazepine, dreaming increases. Immediately after the withdrawal of benzodiazepines, there may be intensification of bizarre dreams. The number of dreams then tends to return to the level prevalent prior to taking the drug (12). The patient's overall medical condition and sleep deprivation due to medical care, as well as the presence of post-traumatic dreams and vivid flashbacks also influence the sleep and dream pattern. The benzodiazepines may diminish anxiety associated with post-traumatic dreams, but we do not know how they affect the pattern.

Benzodiazepines should not be given to patients with sleep apnea; they worsen this condition.

As previously noted, sedating antihistamines and tricyclic antidepressants may be useful in insomnia. The latter group may be particularly useful, especially during the later phase of hospitalization or on an outpatient basis, when hypnotics are unsuccessful in relieving persistent insomnia or a reversed sleep cycle. Titrating the dosage of the tricyclic antidepressant with the previously described precautions can often achieve a good result for sleep difficulties.

ADVERSE EFFECTS

As mentioned, CNS depression is one of the most common side effects of the benzodiazepines. This can present as a generalized sedation and drowsiness or as dysarthric speech, muscle weakness, and nystagmus. There can be paradoxical agitation related to the disinhibiting effect of the benzodiazepines. When this occurs, there may be increased agitation and violent behavior (13). Occasionally, insomnia, nightmares, and even hallucinations are side effects of the benzodiazepines. There can be mild anticholinergic effects that might cause blurred vision. Older patients are more prone to all of these adverse reactions so their dosage should be raised slowly.

As noted above, the long-acting benzodiazepines are more likely to cause prolonged sedation. Anterograde memory impairment has been observed in the clinical use of a variety of benzodiazepines, especially in the short-acting drugs such as lorazepam and alprazolam (14). The ultra-short-acting drug triazolam has been reported to cause episodes of confusion, dissociation, and anterograde amnesia.

The benzodiazepines can cause a decreased CO_2 response and, thus, worsen sleep apnea and other obstructive pulmonary disorders. Such effects become of greater concern when narcotics that depress respiration are also given. The concern lessens when the patient is on a ventilator.

ADMINISTRATION

All benzodiazepines are well absorbed from the gastrointestinal tract after oral administration. Lorazepam is most adequately absorbed via intramuscular administration. Intramuscular chlordiazepoxide and diazepam have slow, erratic absorption, and the injections may cause local pain. Similarly, the I.V. administration of diazepam and chlordiazepoxide can cause local pain and thrombophlebitis due to precipitation or to an irritant effect of propylene glycol (15). Intravenous lorazepam is usually tolerated well. Lorazepam given sublingually has a relatively rapid onset of action (4).

SPECIAL CONSIDERATIONS

Liver Failure

For the most part, benzodiazepines are metabolized in the liver. In patients with cirrhosis of the liver, metabolic liver damage, or active hepatitis, those benzodiazepines that are metabolized by conjugation—for example, oxazepam, lorazepam, and temazepam—are preferable to those metabolized by oxidation (4).

Renal Failure

Although the benzodiazepines are known to be metabolized by the liver into pharmacologically active and inactive metabolites, the elimination of these metabolites is not fully understood. It is believed that several of the benzodiazepines, such as chlorazepate, diazepam, and flurazepam have active metabolites that carry the potential for problems of metabolic accumulation in patients with renal failure. It is, therefore, advisable that lorazepam, oxazepam, or temazepam, all of which have inactive metabolites, be the drugs of choice for such patients (16).

With advanced renal failure, there is less protein binding and, therefore, a greater availability of unbound drugs. This can lead to toxicity or enhanced therapeutic effect for a given dose compared with patients with normal kidney function. It is, therefore, suggested that, with patients who have renal failure, the maximum dose be about one-third less than with patients who have normal renal function (17). Dosage is always titrated against symptoms and side effects.

Benzodiazepines are not dialyzable and, therefore, will not be removed by the process of dialysis (16).

Pulmonary Disease

Benzodiazepines may suppress the hypoxic respiratory drive, placing some pulmonary patients with hypoventilation at risk of respiratory failure. Benzodiazepines should be avoided in patients who chronically retain CO_2, and they are contraindicated in patients with sleep apnea (4). All of these respiratory effects can be intensified if patients are simultaneously receiving narcotics that also suppress respiration.

It is recognized that patients who are dyspnic are often anxious and might benefit from anxiolytic medication. If benzodiazepines are considered at all, blood gases must be carefully monitored while the medication is titrated. There is less concern about respiratory failure if the patient is on a ventilator. In this case, low doses of neuroleptics may also be used, and it has been suggested recently that the antianxiety agent buspirone may have stimulatory effects on respiratory drive (18).

Dependency and Withdrawal

Physical withdrawal symptoms have occurred following abrupt discontinuation of benzodiazepines, ranging from mild dysphoria and insomnia to a major syndrome that can include abdominal and other muscle cramps, vomiting, sweating, tremor, and convulsions. In addition, withdrawal symptoms and even seizures can occur when the dosage is decreased rapidly. With all benzodiazepines, more severe withdrawal usually occurs in patients who have received a high-range dosage over an extended period of time. However, some withdrawal symptoms may occur in some patients even several days after a therapeutic dosage has been stopped, especially with the shorter-acting benzodiazepines.

After an extended dosage and when feasible, a gradual tapering schedule should be followed if a decision to discontinue benzodiazepines has been made.

If a patient enters a hospital following trauma, and has a history of chronic benzodiazepine use, there should not be an abrupt cessation of the medication. If there is a valid therapeutic reason, the benzodiazepine may be continued. Otherwise, it should be appropriately tapered. One suggested technique for reducing extended benzodiazepine usage over a long period is to switch the patient to an equivalent dose of diazepam and to reduce it by 10 mg/day until a dose of 20 mg/day is reached. It then should be reduced 5 mg daily to zero. Propanolol may be helpful in minimizing some withdrawal symptoms (19).

The above method is not effective for alprazolam, which usually must be decreased by 0.5 mg weekly (19) and sometimes even more slowly to avoid withdrawal symptoms. Another technique with all benzodiazepines is to substitute an equivalent dose of the high-potency, long-acting clonazepam, which is usually given twice a day and gradually reduced over a 6- to 8-week period (20).

When benzodiazepines are discontinued, even without full-blown withdrawal symptoms, there can be a recurrence of the original symptoms at a greater intensity than that experienced prior to the onset of the treatment. Rebound can occur when benzodiazepines are used for anxiety, sleep, or other reasons. The rebound phenomena usually last only a few days, and are self-limited. They can be minimized by a small, tapering dosage of the benzodiazepine being withdrawn. The persistence of symptoms suggests an underlying condition that requires treatment. The condition may require continued psychopharmacological treatment, but the need for psychotherapeutic support should also be determined.

On the basis of our discussion of withdrawal above, it is obvious that cessation of benzodiazepine medication should not be abrupt. As we mentioned in the chapter on pain medication, the decision to discharge a burn and trauma patient from the hospital is often made precipitously on medical, surgical, and other grounds, and without taking into account current medications. If the patient will be tapering benzodiazepines as an outpatient, there should be very clear instructions about the plan and the reasons for it. There should also be adequate monitoring of the patient during this period.

On returning home, unanticipated stresses on the patient may lead to the taking of additional benzodiazepines, possibly causing the patient to run out of pills abruptly before a follow-up appointment. This situation could lead to uncomfortable and even dangerous consequences. On the other hand, a reliable patient will follow instructions and contact the doctor if a problem occurs.

Patients with histories of alcohol or substance abuse of any kind, including patients who have misused prescribed medications in the past, are not good candidates for outpatient treatment with benzodiazepines. In such a situation, a trial of buspirone (see below) should be considered for anxiety symptoms. Also, the use of tricyclics, although they are primarily antidepressives, has been effective in treating panic disorder as well as symptoms of post-traumatic stress disorder, and may be especially indicated in this patient group. As with all patients, careful follow-up is important.

PREGNANCY AND THE BENZODIAZEPINES

Although data are inconclusive, some studies suggest an association between benzodiazepines and teratogenicity. High doses of benzodiazepines for a prolonged period in a near-term pregnant woman can cause a withdrawal reaction in the newborn. Benzodiazepines excreted into the breast milk of nursing women may also affect the newborn.

Miscellaneous Anxiolytics

BUSPIRONE

Buspar (buspirone) is a new antianxiety drug that is structurally and pharmacologically unrelated to the benzodiazepines. It is not a central nervous system depressant and does not produce sedative action, as the benzodiazepines do. Buspirone does not cross-react with the benzodiazepines, will not protect against benzodiazepine withdrawals, and does not appear to produce tolerance or dependency. Thus, buspirone may be effective without the risk of dependence. Also, unlike the benzodiazepines, buspirone has no anticonvulsive or muscle-relaxing properties (11).

When used for anxiolytic effect, buspirone must be given regularly (three times a day in the usual dosage range of 15–30 mg/day). Sometimes, a greater amount is given. At least a full 2 weeks of treatment are usually necessary to relieve anxiety; the benzodiazepines often achieve results in a few hours. Often, patients and staff do not have the patience to try this medication, especially if they have recently tried the benzodiazepines or if these drugs are readily available. A possible added advantage of buspirone in a trauma or burn patient is recent evidence that suggests a stimulating effect on respiratory drive.

Other Drugs

β-BLOCKERS

β-Adrenergic blocking drugs, such as propranolol, atenolol, and others, can inhibit physiological manifestations of anxiety if used alone or with a benzodiazepine. These drugs do not usually produce sedation.

PARALDEHYDE

Occasionally, if benzodiazepines and antipsychotic medications cannot be used or are ineffective in controlling an agitated patient, paraldehyde, a rapid-acting hypnotic similar to chloral hydrate, can be used.

A 30-cc oral dose of paraldehyde quietens patients and induces sleep; 10 cc I.M. is also effective, with occasional repetition of 10 cc after the first hour.

The liver metabolizes 70–80% of the above dosages of paraldehyde, and 11–28% is exhaled by the lungs. This leads to a detectable alcohol-like odor in the room of the patient given this substance. Paraldehyde can irritate mucus membranes and cause gastritis. Other sedating drugs, such as the antipsychotics and benzodiazepines, should be avoided within 3 hours of the use of paraldehyde (21).

Antipsychotic Drugs

Antipsychotic drugs are also known as major tranquilizers or neuroleptics. This group of medications is indicated for the acute treatment and maintenance therapy of schizophrenia and for the acute treatment of mania in a patient who has been started on lithium therapy but who has not yet responded to the treatment. Antipsychotic chemotherapy can be useful in other psychotic disorders, including depressive illnesses with psychotic manifestations. In addition, these drugs are useful for conditions accompanied by severe anxiety and agitation.

The major therapeutic effects of these drugs occur during use for acute psychosis. They include the reduction of so-called "positive" symptoms such as hallucinations, delusions, uncooperativeness, and thought disorders, and the normalization of psychomotor activity (excitement or retardation) (22).

While the positive symptoms of a patient with schizophrenia respond consistently to antipsychotic drugs, the "negative" or deficit symptoms— affect flattening, apathy, anhedonia, and thought blocking—are less responsive to them. More recent research reports that the new drug clozapine (Clozaril) is effective in patients with these latter symptoms (23). Because of its adverse effects on bone marrow and an increased risk that it may cause seizures, clozapine must be used with care.

In general, antipsychotic drugs are important for the burn and trauma patient as adjunctive treatments for organic mental syndromes and organic mental disorders, especially in the presence of delirium. The antipsychotic drugs are also useful in the surgical setting as adjuncts to anesthesia or as antiemetics and antipruritics, and for refractory hiccups (21).

Patients with a pre-existing condition that requires antipsychotic medication may suddenly need care in a burn or trauma center after being injured. The decision to continue the patient's previous treatment plan with antipsychotic drugs should be based on the patient's current medical condition, expected hospital course (including possible surgery), and whether the patient's psychiatric history suggests that he or she may suffer acute psychotic symptoms and agitation after termination of the medications. There are usually no significant acute drug withdrawal symptoms when an antipsychotic is stopped. Occasionally, abrupt discontinuation of antipsychotic chemotherapy may provoke a withdrawal dyskinesia (24). In that situation, gradual tapering off of the medication is appropriate.

Synergistic action and drug interactions with other medication, especially when the other drugs are narcotics required for pain control, should be evaluated. Hypotension and sedation are two common effects of antipsychotics and of narcotic drugs. The patient's overall medical condition and the life-threatening injuries that led to hospitalization and perhaps critical care should be of primary importance. If there is doubt, the antipsychotic medication can be withheld. If psychotic decompensation occurs, it usually develops gradually. Because acute burn and trauma patients are usually under close scrutiny in the hospital, antipsychotic drugs can be reinstituted if symptoms appear. Response to medication will usually occur within hours or days. If the patient's medical condition and treatment do not have possible contraindications, antipsychotic drugs can be continued while the patient receives medical and surgical treatment.

A person who may have had a psychotic decompensation that caused behavior that subsequently led to an accident with serious injury and hospitalization, may require immediate antipsychotic medication as well as immediate treatment for the injury. This may be the first time that the individual has been diagnosed as having a psychotic condition.

Perhaps a person who had been treated for psychosis stopped the antipsychotic and now requires a reinstitution of drugs. A patient with an organic mental syndrome of known or unknown cause requires psychopharmacological intervention. The patient may be wandering, agitated, combative, assaultive, screaming, paranoid, or have other delusions.

A diagnostic distinction should be made between the acute organic picture occurring after the burn or trauma injury, and a pre-existing or underlying organic brain disorder that is more common in but not limited to elderly patients. The psychopharmacological approach may be the same in both cases. Antipsychotic drugs have been the traditional psychopharmacological approach to disturbances of behavior and thinking that arise from organic mental disorders or that are due to underlying or coexisting nonorganic psychotic disorders. These medications are appropriate to treat related behavioral symptoms, although neither exclusively nor in all situations.

Antipsychotic drugs have several advantages over benzodiazepines. First, they decrease psychotic psychomotor activity and flatten affect without producing significant sedation or stupor, which inhibits patient cooperation during care. Second, the antipsychotic drugs do not produce tolerance to their effects and do not produce physical dependence. Third, even high doses of the drugs given to produce somnolence do not cause complete immobility. Total immobility may lead to decubiti, phlebothrombosis, pulmonary embolism, or bronchopneumonia (25).

Potential disadvantages of the antipsychotic medications in the burn and trauma setting are the three kinds of side effects that are potentially troublesome for the medically compromised patient in general. These side

effects—sedation, orthostatic hypotension, and extrapyramidal symptoms—
are discussed below. In addition, it should be noted that antipsychotics are
useless for the prevention of alcohol withdrawal symptoms. Antipsychotics
differ pharmacologically from alcohol and sedatives. They could be potentially harmful in that situation because they lower the seizure threshold.
Treatment of alcohol withdrawal is discussed in a later chapter.

When control of dangerous behavior is desired within minutes, short-
acting benzodiazepines are usually used, occasionally with short-acting barbiturates. Consideration should be given to switching over to antipsychotic
drugs to avoid physical dependence and withdrawal symptoms, which can
occur on sudden abstinence after 10 days to 2 weeks. Such a consideration
is particularly relevant to the large doses of benzodiazepines necessary to
control violent or severely agitated behavior. As described, the benzodiazepines may cause additional problems in the medical setting by depressing
respiration. Sometimes, the combination of a benzodiazepine and an antipsychotic drug can control extreme agitation.

Regarding efficacy, no one antipsychotic drug is consistently superior to
another. They are equally effective at optimal doses (22). Some patients
respond better to one drug than another, but only previous history of a good
response is a reliable predictor.

The various antipsychotic drugs differ from each other in potency and in
selectivity with respect to the postsynaptic dopamine receptor blockade,
their presumed mode of action. Therefore, differences in the various antipsychotic drugs relate to their side effects.

As a rule, the low potency drugs produce more sedation, more orthostatic
hypotension, and more anticholinergic effects. The high potency agents produce more frequent and more severe extrapyramidal symptoms (see Table
6.3). The significance of these symptoms, especially as they concern the
burn and trauma patient, will be discussed below.

Generally, because of the existing high potential for cerebral dysfunction
in medically compromised burn and trauma patients due to the confluence
of such forces as other medications, electrolyte disturbance, unstable blood
pressure, shifting fluid volume, and concurrent infection, high-potency
antipsychotics are the drug of choice when this class of drug is needed (26).
This is especially true in the elderly, who have increased sensitivity to the
effects and side effects of the drug.

ADMINISTRATION

Most antipsychotic medications are in liquid as well as pill form. If possible, this medication should not be given within 2 hours of an antacid or

Table 6.3 Commonly Used Antipsychotics[a]

	Approximately Equivalent Dosage (mg)	Relative Potency	Usual Daily Dosage Range (mg)	Anticholinergic Effects Observed Clinically	Parkinsonian Effects Observed Clinically	Sedation Effects Observed Clinically	Hypotensive Effects Observed Clinically
Phenothiazines							
Aliphatic							
Chlorpromazine[b,c] (Thorazine)	100	Low	30–800	+ + + +	+ +	+ + + + +	+ + + + +
Piperidine							
Mesoridazine (Serentil)	75	Medium	25–400	+ + +	+ + +	+ + + +	+ + + +
Thioridazine (Mellaril)	100	Low	30–400	+ + + + +	+	+ + + +	+ + + + +
Piperazine							
Fluphenazine[b] (Prolixin)	2	High	4–20	+ +	+ + + + +	+ +	+ +
Perphenazine[b] (Trilafon)	10	Medium	4–24	+ +	+ + + +	+ + +	+ + +
Trifluoperazine (Stelazine)	5	High	2–40	+ +	+ + + +	+	+ +
Thioxanthene							
Thiothixene[b] (Navane)	3	High	6–60	+ +	+ + + +	+ +	+ +
Butyrophenone							
Haloperidol[b] (Haldol)	2	High	1–100	+	+ + + + +	+ +	+
Dibenzoxazepine							
Loxapine (Loxitane)	15	Medium	10–100	+ +	+ + +	+ + +	+ +
Dihydroindolone							
Molindone (Moban)	10	Medium	15–225	+ +	+ + +	+	+ +

[a] This table is based on a composite of various published studies and charts (21, 22, 24) and our own clinical experience.
[b] Available parenteral dosage.
[c] Available in rectal suppository.

antidiarrheal; both decrease absorption of the drug. Some liquids, such as chlorpromazine, have a local anesthetic effect and should be well diluted to prevent choking (21).

If medication is given I.M., the patient should be kept supine or seated for a half hour to avoid orthostatic hypotension. The blood pressure can be monitored before and after each injection. Several antipsychotic drugs come in slow release, long-lasting depot form, with a duration of 2–4 weeks. These forms are unusual for the treatment of acute burn and trauma patients. However, if patients entered the hospital with such medication on board, it is important to observe the effects of such drugs.

If oral and parenteral sites are inappropriate, chlorpromazine rectal suppositories are available. This drug, whose action is similar to that of a prochlorperazine suppository, is used occasionally as an antiemetic.

Antipsychotics are yet unapproved for I.V. use by the FDA. However, I.V. haloperidol has been reported to be safe and effective within 30 minutes (27). It is often given in I.V. form in emergency situations for extreme agitation or psychosis. Under these circumstances, it is the drug of choice for the medically ill patient. It has little or no anticholinergic or hypotensive effect, and does not usually oversedate or cause respiratory depression. The starting dose of I.V. haloperidol is 0.5–2.0 mg. The I.V. dosage is half the oral dosage. For more severely agitated patients, a starting dose of 2.0–5.0 mg can be used. The I.V. line should be cleared with normal saline before bolus infusion, allowing 30 minutes between doses. With continued agitation, the previous dosage can be doubled. Lorazepam (Ativan) is often combined with haloperidol in difficult cases. Lorazepam I.V. (0.5–1.0 mg) can be given concurrently or alternatingly with haloperidol every 30 minutes. When the patient is calm, the total dosage of the haloperidol administered to achieve that state can be given over the next 24 hours. When the patient is stable, the dosage should be tapered by a 50% reduction every 24 hours (28, 29).

SIDE EFFECTS

The following are some side effects of antipsychotic medications that may be particularly pertinent to the burn and trauma patient. The treating physician as well as the psychiatric consultants and nurses should be familiar with the complete *PDR* description and package inserts of any prescribed drug.

Cardiovascular

The phenothiazine antipsychotic drugs, particularly the low-potency agents such as thioridazine (Mellaril) and chlorpromazine (Thorazine), can cause prolongation of cardiac conduction time and lead to prolonged PR and QTc intervals on the electrocardiogram, both of which are usually of minor significance unless the patient is also taking a Type I antiarrhythmia drug and/or has a significant pre-existing heart block (26).

Patients who have a rare pre-existing QTc syndrome (QT interval greater than 0.440 seconds) may develop a fatal ventricular tachycardia with drugs, including the tricyclics, that cause a quinidine-like effect. Thioridazine appears to be the phenothiazine most commonly associated with this syndrome (26, 30).

Orthostatic hypotension is a potentially serious side effect that can occur with antipsychotic drugs, but it is less likely with the high-potency drugs. Haloperidol (Haldol), which has the least α-adrenergic blocking effect, is least likely among the antipsychotics to induce hypotension. It should be particularly noted that chlorpromazine (Thorazine), mesoridazine (Serentil), and thioridazine (Mellaril) each can cause considerable hypotension if used alone. All three can be especially dangerous if combined with coronary, cerebral, or peripheral vasodilators or with antihypertensive drugs whose hypotensive effects intensify. The combination of phenothiazines and the MAO inhibitor antidepressive drugs can also cause severe hypotension (31).

Patients receiving medications that cause orthostatic hypotension should be cautioned about getting up rapidly to avoid falls and injuries.

Persistent hypotension from these drug interactions is best treated by keeping the patient in a recumbent position, providing I.V. fluid replacements through a large catheter, and monitoring the patient carefully to avoid congestive heart failure. If a pressor agent is necessary, phenylephrine is the safest but should be used cautiously. Epinephrine should be avoided; its β-adrenergic stimulant effect may induce further hypotension (30). When phenothiazines combine with a variety of anesthetics, such as halothane, enflurane, and isoflurane, there is considerable likelihood of hypotensive reactions (30, 32).

Anticholinergic

The possible anticholinergic effects of antipsychotic medications are blurred vision, dry mouth, tachycardia, constipation, and urinary retention. These medications may also affect the central nervous system and produce stuttering, impaired memory, difficulty with concentration, and, in rare cases, a delirium. Patients who receive antipsychotic drugs may also be receiving antiparkinsonian drugs and perhaps tricyclic antidepressants, which can intensify the cholinergic blockade. Any other drugs with anticholinergic properties add to this problem.

Urinary retention may be managed with bethanechol but, if persistent, may require a change in medication. Laxatives and stool softeners may relieve constipation that occurs because of the anticholinergic effect.

Sedation

Antipsychotic drugs in low initial doses and then in progressively incremental doses to the point of sleepiness with arousability, produce the equivalent of normal sleep (25). Untoward sedative effects will not usually occur unless a drug such as benzodiazepine or a narcotic is added to the antipsychotic. Such a drug further depresses the patient's level of consciousness and respiratory center, particularly if the patient has an underlying chronic obstructive pulmonary disease or is elderly (24, 31). Sedation occurs most commonly with the low-potency antipsychotics.

Extrapyramidal Symptoms

Extrapyramidal symptoms are important side effects of antipsychotic drugs. These may occur immediately after the onset of treatment or insidiously over the first month and may be due to the nigrostriatal dopamine blockade. The cessation of the antipsychotic medication, reduction in dosage, or switch to a low-potency agent can all be effective treatments for these symptoms, as is the addition of antiparkinsonian drugs described below.

Three kinds of extrapyramidal effects can occur. The first group are the *dystonias*, which include torsions, twistings, and the drawing of muscle groups, causing painful muscle spasms. These usually occur within a few days of beginning the medication. Prominent among these symptoms are the oculogyric crises characterized by a rolling up of the eyes. Young men are at greatest risk for this group of symptoms.

Diphenhydramine (Benadryl), 25–50 mg I.V., provides the most rapid—within minutes—and safe relief. Alternatively, diphenhydramine I.M. or benzotropine (Cogentin) I.V. or I.M. (1–2 mg) may be given (24). Oral antiparkinsonians are also useful, but do not achieve as rapid a result as the I.M. form. A benzodiazepine such as sublingual lorazepam (Ativan) can also achieve fast relief. Other antiparkinsonians used to treat these symptoms include biperiden (Akineton), trihexyphenidyl (Artane), amatidine (Symmetrel), orphenedrine (Disipal), procyclidine (Kemadrin), and ethopropazine (Parsidol).

Akathisia, a motor restlessness sometimes called "restless legs," is a more common reaction to antipsychotics. The reaction can be a generalized motor or mental restlessness. It usually occurs within the first 10 days of administration of the antipsychotic, and can affect 12–45% of patients on these drugs. Elderly women have the highest risk of this side effect. The treatment of choice for akathisia is an oral antiparkinsonian described above, but oral diazepam (Valium) or β blockers, such as propranolol and nadolol, have been used (21).

The third category of extrapyramidal effects of antipsychotics is the pseudoparkinsonian group of symptoms—stiffness, shuffling, masklike facies, tremors, akathisia, and rigidity or cogwheeling of the limbs. This complex of symptoms may occur within the first 30 days of the administration of antipsychotics in 12–45% of the population. Again, oral antiparkinsonians are the treatment of choice.

Although prophylactic administration of an antiparkinsonian drug in low dosage (two to four times/day) may reduce the incidence and severity of acute extrapyramidal symptoms, it can cause additional problems in the elderly or in patients with organic mental syndrome due to its anticholinergic and sedative side effects. If antipsychotic medication is required despite extrapyramidal side effects, the first choice should be low-potency drugs.

After months or years of treatment with antipsychotic medication, patients can develop tardive dyskinesia, which may even continue after discontinuation of the drugs. Symptoms include repetitive lip smacking, masticatory and tongue movements, and choreic movements of the trunk and limbs. The cause is believed to be long-term chronic blockade of postsynaptic receptors, which results in denervation supersensitivity of the striatal tracks of the basal ganglia (24). All of the standard antipsychotic drugs may produce tardive dyskinesia in approximately 20% of the patients receiving prolonged treatment. One exception appears to be the new antipsychotic clozapine (Clozaril).

Lower doses or short-term administration of antipsychotics may reduce the risk of tardive dyskinesia. Tardive dyskinesia often diminishes and disappears after a prolonged drug-free interval. Clonadine, cholinesterase inhibitors, and cholinergic precursors are often useful in the treatment of tardive dyskinesia. The possibility of tardive dyskinesia enters into the decision of whether or not to keep a burn and trauma patient on an antipsychotic medication after successful treatment for symptoms, usually during an early phase of treatment. In most cases, with symptoms in remission, we attempt to manage the patient without antipsychotic drugs, unless there is a history of the patient developing psychotic symptoms when taken off this medication.

Seizure Thresholds

Antipsychotic drugs lower seizure thresholds and should be used with caution in patients with a history of seizures. This effect has been reported most frequently with chlorpromazine (Thorazine) and the new antipsychotic clozapine (Clozaril). Among the less potent agents, thioridazine (Mellaril) and mesoridazine (Serentil) seem less proconvulsant than chlorpromazine. In vitro work suggests that molindone (Moban) and fluphenazine (Prolixin) may have the least effect on seizure threshold (26). Because antipsychotic drugs may affect anticonvulsant blood levels, these should be monitored during the initiation of the drugs (26).

Neuroleptic Malignant Syndrome

Neuroleptic malignant syndrome (NMS) is a rare (less than 1%), potentially fatal reaction in patients receiving antipsychotic medication. It occurs after initiating or increasing this medication. Dehydrated, medically debilitated, and neurologically impaired patients are at somewhat higher risk for this syndrome. Males are affected twice as often as females, and 80% of reported patients have been under age 40 years.

Patients with NMS have muscular rigidity with akinesia and, often, a catatonic appearance. There is hyperthermia (the temperature may range from 101–106°F), and consciousness is altered. The patient may be alert, show "dazed mutism" or stupor, or be comatose. Profound autonomic dysfunction with labile blood pressure, profuse diaphoresis, sialorrhea, incontinence, and dysphasia accompany NMS. There is also elevated blood CPK.

Neuroleptic malignant syndrome is a medical emergency; antipsychotic medication must be stopped *immediately*. Adequate oral or I.V. hydration with a correction of electrolyte abnormalities and symptomatic management of fever is necessary. Medical consultations should be obtained. Bromocriptine (up to 60 mg/day) or dantrolene (200 mg/day) may be beneficial in severe NMS (22, 33).

Hematological

Antipsychotic drugs can cause a benign leukopenia, thrombocytopenia, or a pancytopenia. The leukopenia is generally not dangerous, usually stabilizing at an approximate white count of 3000. Agranulocytosis, a much more serious side effect, has an incidence of 1 in 500,000 and occurs abruptly less than 8 weeks after the start of treatment. Chlorpromazine (Thorazine) is most frequently indicated in this complication. Because hospitalized patients have periodic blood counts, this potential adverse effect can be monitored in the hospitalized burn and trauma patient. Symptoms of agranulocytosis include sore throat and fever (22, 33). The new antipsychotic clozapine (Clozaril) reportedly has an incidence of agranulocytosis that is as high as 1–2% (26).

Liver

Transient elevation of liver function tests in patients on antipsychotics, especially chlorpromazine (Thorazine), usually do not indicate the onset of severe toxicity (26), nor the need for cessation of the medication as a consequence.

Cholestatic jaundice occurs within the first 4 weeks of treatment in less than 0.1% of the patients on antipsychotic drugs. Signs include yellow skin, dark urine, and pruritus. It is reversible if the drug is stopped (21). Antipsychotic drugs should be used with caution in patients with severe liver disease.

Pulmonary

Head-injured patients may suffer significant respiratory depression with antipsychotic medications (34). Patients with chronic pulmonary disease who are placed on antipsychotics may develop abnormal involuntary movements in the respiratory musculature that are experienced as dyspnea (26).

Endocrine

Endocrine effects, including moderate breast engorgement, lactation, amenorrhea, false positive pregnancy tests, menstrual irregularities, and changes in libido in women, can occur.

Inhibition of ejaculation, loss of libido, and gynecomastia are possible in men taking antipsychotic drugs. Prostatism can be exacerbated, especially by low potency antipsychotic drugs (26).

Hypoglycemia, hyperglycemia, and increased appetite or increased weight are also associated with these drugs.

Eye Changes

Pigmentary retinopathy, primarily associated with the use of thioridazine (Mellaril) and chlorpromazine (Thorazine), can occur. Potential exists for an exacerbation of narrow angle glaucoma, especially in patients with this condition who are treated with antipsychotic drugs that have increased anticholinergic effect (26).

End-Stage Renal Disease

Antipsychotic drugs are lipid soluble and are excreted by the kidneys. Their elimination is by liver biotransformation to inactive metabolites that are excreted. Decreased drug concentration is possible in patients who have renal failure due to diminished protein-binding ability. Antipsychotic medications may be used in patients with renal failure, but a smaller dosage than usual is appropriate in patients with renal failure due to the above reasons (16).

OTHER SIDE EFFECTS

Due to inhibition of the hypothalamic control areas, the use of antipsychotics can alter the ability of the body to regulate the response to changes in temperature and humidity. This can lead to hyperthermia or hypothermia. The use of moderate to high doses of antipsychotics in the last trimester of pregnancy may produce extrapyramidal reactions in newborns and impaired temperature regulation after birth. Whether these drugs have teratogenetic effects is unclear. As with all drugs, their use should be avoided during the first trimester if possible (21).

Lithium

Lithium therapy is an established treatment for acute mania and for prophylaxis against recurrent mania in major affective disorders—bipolar type. It has also often been used jointly with other antidepressant medications as a mood stabilizer in the treatment of depression and, at times, for other psychiatric conditions. Blood lithium levels are monitored in the course of treatment with lithium. The usual level used for acute mania is 1.0–1.5 mEq/L, with 0.6–1.2 mEq/L as the level for maintenance.

There must be sufficient renal function to prevent a dangerous buildup of lithium. Sodium depletion or other electrolyte imbalances, such as those brought about by sodium restricted diets, diuretics, blood loss, I.V. infusion, fluid shifts, and shock can all cause potential lithium toxicity. A person who is lithium toxic can develop cardiac arrhythymia, impaired consciousness, muscle fasciculations, hyperreflexia, nystagmus, convulsions, coma, oliguria, and anuria. Lithium toxicity can cause death.

Many of the conditions that can lead to lithium toxicity can be present during the acute phase of a burn or trauma injury. It is for this reason that we do not advise the continuation or institution of lithium administration during the acute phase of an injury and the initial period of hospitalization. There is no withdrawal syndrome with the abrupt cessation of lithium. It is unlikely that a patient on maintenance lithium will develop an immediate acute manic episode.

If a person was injured during an acute manic episode, the initial narcotics given for pain control will sedate the patient. If the patient is having acute psychotic manic symptoms, an antipsychotic drug, such as haloperidol or others described earlier in this chapter, can be given. Once the patient has been medically stabilized, the use of lithium can be considered if clinically appropriate. When using lithium, drug interactions with other drugs being given must be carefully taken into account as should its effect on various organ systems that may be compromised (35).

Two anticonvulsants, carbamazepine (Tegretol) and sodium valproate, have also been used in the treatment of mania as an alternative to lithium. These drugs also require close monitoring with blood levels, CBC, and liver function tests (36).

References

1. Physicians' desk reference. 43rd ed. Oradell, NJ: Medical Economics, 1989:2060–2061.
2. Rabkin J, Quitkin F, McGrath P, et al. Adverse reactions to monoamine oxidase inhibitors. II. Treatment correlates and clinical management. J Clin Psychopharmacol 1985;5:2–9.
3. Muskin PR, Glassman AH, Alexander H. The use of tricyclic antidepressants in a medical setting. In: Finkel J, ed. Consultation/liaison. Current trends and perspectives. New York: Grune & Stratton, 1983:137–158.
4. Stoudemire A, Moran MG, Fogel S, et al. Psychotropic drug use in the medically ill. Part I. Psychosomatics 1990;31:377–392.
5. Bigger JT, Giardina EGV, Perel JM, et al. Cardiac antiarrhythmic effect of imipramine hydrochloride. N Engl J Med 1977;296:206–208.
6. Edwards JG, Long SK, Sedgwick EM, et al. Antidepressants and convulsive seizures: clinical electroencephalographic and pharmacological aspects. Clin Neuropharmacol 1986;9:329–360.
7. Davidson J. Seizures and bupropion: a review. J Clin Psychiatry 1989;50:256–261.
8. Regier DA, Narrow WE, Rae DS. The epidemiology of anxiety disorders: the epidemiologic catchment area experience. J Psychiatr Res 1990;24:3–14.
9. Kaplan H, Sadock B. Pocket handbook of clinical psychiatry. Baltimore: Williams & Wilkins, 1990:230–270.
10. Derogatis LR, Wise TN. Treatment of anxiety state and depressive disorders in the medical patient. In: Anxiety and depression in the medical patient. Washington: American Psychiatric Press, 1989:199–257.
11. Bernstein JG. Antianxiety agents and hypnotics. In: Handbook of drug therapy in psychiatry. 2nd ed. Littleton, MA: PSG Publishing, Inc., 1988:51–77.
12. Kales A, Solsatos, Kales JD. Sleep disorders: Insomnia, sleep walking, night terror, and enuresis. Ann Intern Med 1987;106:582–592.

13. Hall RCW, Zisook S. Paradoxical reactions to benzodiazepines. Br J Clin Pharmacol 1981; 11:995–1015.
14. Kumar R, Mac DS, Gabrielli WF, et al. Anxiolytics and memory. A comparison of lorazepam and alprazolam. J Clin Psychiatry 1987;48:158–160.
15. Reading AE. Testing pain mechanisms in pain. In: Wall PD, Melzack R, eds. Textbook of pain. 2nd ed. Edinburgh: Churchill Livingstone, 1989:269–280.
16. Levy NB. Psychopharmacology in patients with renal failure. Int J Psychiatry Med 1990; 20:303–312.
17. Levy NB. Use of psychotropics in patients with kidney failure. Psychosomatics 1985;26:699–709.
18. Garner SJ, Eldridge FL, Wagner PG, et al. Buspirone, an anxiolytic drug that stimulates respiration. Am Rev Respir Dis 1989;139:946–950.
19. Bezchlibnyk-Butler KZ, Jeffries JJ, ed. Clinical handbook of psychotropic drugs. 2nd ed. Toronto: Hogrefe & Huber, 1990:31–39.
20. DuPont RJ. A practical approach to benzodiazepines. J Psychiatr Res 1990;24:81–90.
21. Bezchlibnyk-Butler KZ, Jeffries JJ, ed. Clinical handbook of psychotropic drugs. 2nd ed. Toronto: Hogrefe & Huber, 1990:12–27.
22. Kaplan HI, Sadock BJ. Organic therapy. In: Pocket handbook of clinical psychiatry. Baltimore: Williams & Wilkins, 1990:230–270.
23. Meltzer HY, Burnett S, Bastini B., et al. Effects of six months of clozapine treatment on the quality of life of chronic schizophrenic patients. Hosp Community Psychiatry 1990;41:892–897.
24. Bernstein JG. Antipsychotic drugs. In: Handbook of drug therapy in psychiatry. 2nd ed. Littleton, MA: PSG Publishing, Inc., 1988:79–121.
25. Glickman L. Psychopharmacology. In: Psychiatric consultation in the general hospital. New York: Marcel Dekker, 1980:205–233.
26. Stoudemire A, Moran MG, Fogel BS. Psychotropic drug use in the medically ill. Psychosomatics 1991;32:34–46.
27. Dudley DL, Rowlett DB, Loebel PJ. Emergency use of intravenous haloperidol. Gen Hosp Psychiatry 1979;1:240–246.
28. Wise M, Cassem NH. Psychiatric consultation to critical-care units. In: Tasman A, Goldfinger SM, Kaufman CA, eds. Review of psychiatry. vol. 9. Washington, DC: American Psychiatric Press, 1990:413–432.
29. Wise MG, Rundell JR. Concise guide to consultation psychiatry. Washington, DC: American Psychiatric Press, 1988:50.
30. Stoudemire A, Fogel BS. Psychopharmacology in the medically ill. In: Stoudemire A, Fogel BS, eds. Principles of medical psychiatry. Orlando, FL: Grune & Stratton, 1987:79–112.
31. Bernstein JC. Drug-drug interaction in the medical setting. In: Haupt JL, Brodie HKH. Psychiatry. vol. 3. Consultation-liaison psychiatry and behavioral medicine. New York: Basic Books, Inc., 1986:297–308.
32. Janowsky EC, Risch C, Janowsky DS. Effect of anesthesia on patients taking psychotropic drugs. J Clin Psychopharmacol 1981;1:14–20.
33. Bernstein JG. Medical complications of psychotropic drugs. In: Handbook of drug therapies in psychiatry. 2nd ed. Littleton, MA: PSG Publishing, Inc., 1988:277–307.
34. Hershey SC, Hales RE. Psychopharmacologic approach to the medically ill patient. Psychiatr Clin North Am 1984;7:803–816.
35. Das Gupta K, Jefferson JJ. The use of lithium in the medically ill. Gen Hosp Psychiatry 1990;12:83–97.
36. Bernstein JG. Lithium and other mood stabilizing drugs. In: Handbook of drug therapy in psychiatry. 2nd ed. Littleton, MA: PSG Publishing, Inc., 1988:207–252.

Alcohol and Substance Abuse

Deadly Connection Between Alcohol and Trauma or Burn

The connection between alcohol and the trauma or burn patient is deadly. Available evidence implicates alcohol consumption as a major risk for almost all kinds of injuries, and there is an exceptionally strong relationship between alcohol and motor vehicle accidents, particularly single-vehicle crashes (1). Alcohol has been involved in 65–70% of fatal highway crashes (2).

During a 6-month period, blood drawn from 615 trauma patients at the University of Texas Medical Center in Dallas showed that 58.9% of the patients had alcohol in their blood. Of that group, 74% had an alcohol level greater than 100 mg/dl (3). A sample of 936 patients admitted to a university trauma center in San Diego had similar results: more than two-thirds of the patients were found to have consumed alcohol (4). In a study of 277 adult patients consecutively hospitalized for burn injuries in New York City, the most common predisposing factors were alcohol and drug abuse, physical and mental illness, and advanced age (5).

A review of eight of nine descriptive studies indicates that exposure to alcohol was more likely among those who died in fires ignited by cigarettes than in fires attributed to other causes (6). In yet another study, after adjustments for severity of burn, statistical increases in mortality were associated with alcohol intake (as well as with certain psychiatric diagnoses) (7). These findings agree with our clinical experience of more than 20 years in city and county hospitals that alcohol intoxication is frequently associated with burn and trauma injuries.

We note an interesting paradox to the expectation that alcohol increases the chances for more severe injury. In an animal study, ethanol ingestion *improved* mean burn severity at 48 hours. Ethanol, acting as a vasodilator, improved dermal circulation and reduced overall extent of injury in this study (8). Even if a high blood alcohol level does protect some individuals from a more severe injury than they might have had, this does not neutralize the role that alcohol may have played in causing the accident.

The alcoholic person who is injured adds trauma to his or her already compromised body. Often, during early phases of alcohol addiction, orthopedic complications, including sprains, fractures, and other injuries occur, because of blackouts or falls (9). Liver failure or malnutrition from chronic alcohol ingestion may seriously impair the body's ability to survive a major injury.

Acute Intoxication

The burn and trauma team in the medical emergency room frequently is the first to treat the acutely intoxicated patient. The patient in this state is often threatening, disruptive, and angry. Hackett believes that the best means of interaction with the acutely intoxicated patient is to accept the "drunk" temporarily as he or she is and to tolerate insults and threats without taking them personally. He advises medical and nursing personnel to listen to such a patient's tirade and to attempt to make some sense of it, rather than demand that the patient lower his or her voice and talk more temperately. Eye contact should be avoided; this is often considered a challenge. The interviewer, according to Hackett, should listen seriously to the patient and appear puzzled or perplexed rather than angry or amused if the accusations the patient makes are absurd. Above all, avoid being belligerent (10).

If medically feasible, it is good to offer the patient food and coffee. Often, if the patients eat, they lose their "fight." If the patient's behavior is frightening, it may be helpful to let the patient know that he or she is frightening staff and other patients. If an immediate procedure is necessary, the patient should be told clearly what is going to be done. Sufficient force should be available to restrain him or her.

As is the case with other patients, the acutely intoxicated patient with a burn or trauma injury requires pain medication. However, the narcotics that may be required for pain and the alcohol present in the body have a synergistic sedating effect on the patient. Therefore, a smaller than usual amount of narcotic is necessary to avoid a deleterious interaction between the alcohol and the pain medication.

Alcohol will, of course, have an anesthetic effect on the patient. Therefore, patients who are intoxicated may not reveal to the staff injuries that they have sustained and often will not experience the amount of pain expected for the severity of the injury.

Benzodiazepines are usually advised for sedation of the intoxicated patient. If parenteral use is required, diazepam (Valium) or lorazepam (Ativan) i.m. or I.V. can be given. Manufacturers' instructions for preparation and administration of I.V. medication should be followed. Because erratic and slow absorption frequently occurs i.m., oral or I.V. use is preferred. The initial dose is usually between 5 and 15 mg of diazepam and between 0.5 and 2.0 mg of lorazepam followed by a wait of 0.5–1.0 hours before repeating the dose if necessary.

Pathological Intoxication

One variant of acute intoxication occurs when individuals become intoxicated with a small amount of alcohol. This state can last for an hour or a few days. The patient in this state may be violent, assaultive, agitated, and aggressive. This disorder is marked by hyperactivity, anxiety, or depression. Sometimes the person may have delusions and visual hallucinations. The episode usually ends after prolonged sleep. If a person has a history of pathological intoxication, he or she should be heavily sedated if possible (10, 11). In addition to pain medication for the injury, benzodiazepines, as previously described, are usually necessary.

Blood Alcohol Level in the Emergency Room

If blood alcohol and drug screens were routine in all trauma and burn patients, more diagnoses of substance abuse would be made and more instances of alcohol withdrawal syndrome, with its possible life-threatening complications, would be prevented.

State laws use varying blood levels to define driving while under the influence or intoxication. This blood level is usually around 0.10% (100 mg/dl). A blood alcohol level of 0.15% (150 mg/dl) is almost always considered pathognomonic for alcoholism (9). Reluctance by staff to take blood alcohol levels may be caused by concern that such evidence could be used against the patient in subsequent liability action or that it would cause insurance problems. Any accident that occurs while drinking may indicate that the person has an alcohol problem and may have underlying psychological problems that led to alcohol use.

In a recent study, 90% of the persons intoxicated at the time of burn injury were found to have a history of alcohol abuse. Only 11% of the nonintoxicated burn patients showed a similar alcohol history (12). Although an intoxicated trauma patient may plead that his or her accident was the result of a single, unfortunate occasion, caregivers should suspect a long-term problem.

Alcohol Withdrawal Syndrome

The recognition of alcohol withdrawal syndrome—delirium tremens—in its full-blown clinical state is quite important because a 10–25% mortality rate usually accompanies untreated delirium tremens (10). The high consumption of alcohol in the U.S. should not be underestimated. It is crucial not to miss diagnosing alcohol withdrawal syndrome in a patient who has a burn or trauma injury.

Alcohol withdrawal usually does not develop in patients under the age of 30 and seldom occurs in patients who have less than 2 years of chronic alcoholism. However, patients who have an alcohol problem frequently underreport their intake and minimize the difficulties they have had with alcohol.

Alcohol withdrawal syndrome may begin in individuals who are still consuming alcohol. It may occur when the person reduces alcohol intake or even when alcohol consumption remains the same because, as tolerance increases, the body requires more alcohol. Of course, if trauma or burn injuries lead to hospitalization, the alcohol intake ceases abruptly.

DIAGNOSES OF ALCOHOL WITHDRAWAL OR DELIRIUM TREMENS

In the earlier stage of alcohol withdrawal, which can begin in the first 12–72 hours after alcohol intake is stopped or relatively diminished, the patient frequently has a loss of appetite, nausea, and irritability. Often, a tremulousness may set in, beginning with a fine tremor and progressing to more severe manifestations. Early on, the patient may report hearing "clicking sounds," seeing a "shimmering screen," or experiencing other mild hallucinations.

The tremor can increase and involve the tongue, rendering the patient unable to speak. The lower extremities may tremble so much that the patient becomes unable to walk. The hands may shake and the patient may become incapable of holding a glass without spilling its contents. Hypervigilance and a characteristic exaggerated startle response also occur, as does frequent marked insomnia.

Grand mal seizures can occur within the first 1 or 2 days after alcohol withdrawal. More than one-third of the patients who have seizures with alcohol withdrawal develop full-blown delirium tremens (10).

The advanced picture of alcohol withdrawal may occur 24–72 hours after the onset of symptoms, especially if there is no treatment. Symptoms include disorientation to time, place, or person, in any combination. The tremor, as previously described, varies from moderate to severe. Hyperactivity is usual. The patient frequently has hallucinations that are visual but can also be tactile, olfactory, or auditory. The hallucinations frighten the patient and can include images of animals, such as snakes, that seem to threaten the patient. Patients see insects or feel them crawling on their skin. Vestibular disturbances can give the patient the feeling that the floor is moving. Increased autonomic arousal is accompanied by fever, sweating, tachycardia, and hypertension.

If untreated, symptoms of alcohol withdrawal can continue for as long as 2 weeks, even without the appearance of full-blown delirium. This persistence of symptoms is an important indicator of alcohol withdrawal because narcotics given for pain or small doses of benzodiazepines given for symptomatic treatment related to the burn or trauma may mask the clinical picture, especially by suppressing autonomic signs of withdrawal. However, there is no cross-tolerance between alcohol and narcotics, and narcotics do not eliminate the potential for a dangerous alcohol withdrawal syndrome.

Alcohol withdrawal should be suspected in any burn or trauma patient who develops a delirium or an organic mental syndrome during the first 7 days of hospitalization. Also, in some patients, alcohol withdrawal syndrome does not appear until 7 days after the last drink. Alcoholics are known to be notoriously inaccurate in reporting their drinking history.

In addition to including alcoholic withdrawal syndrome, the differential diagnosis of delirium or organic mental syndrome in the burn and trauma patient should include other substance abuse or drug withdrawal, postconcussion head injury, or metabolic disorders—including impending hepatic coma and acute pancreatitis (10). Delirium secondary to narcotics or other medications, medical conditions such as degenerative brain disorders, and tumors and infections—including HIV (human immunodeficiency virus)—should be considered in a differential diagnosis or as a coexisting condition.

TREATMENT OF ALCOHOL WITHDRAWAL AND DELIRIUM TREMENS

The patients going through withdrawal must be closely watched so that they cannot hurt themselves or others. This usually requires around-the-clock nursing care. Restraints, if needed, should be used for short periods, and the patients must be relieved from them at least every 2 hours.

Proper hydration is essential and electrolyte imbalance must be corrected. Except in mild cases, I.V. therapy is a usual requirement for the treatment of alcohol withdrawal syndrome. In patients with burn injury, this aspect of treatment is closely monitored by the medical/surgical treatment teams. Fluid management during the resuscitation phase of burn injury is important. This is also relevant with significant trauma injury. One study of accident victims suggests that patients who suffer from delirium tremens have low serum potassium levels (13).

Potential problems can also occur in patients with simple trauma. Preliminary treatment, such as fracture reduction and casting, may be done without I.V. treatment and close observation and follow-up. In such situations, a serious alcohol withdrawal syndrome may develop and remain undetected.

The cornerstone treatment of alcohol withdrawal is the administration of a drug that sedates the patient and prevents full-blown delirium tremens. The most common drug and the one we recommend for that use is chlordiazepoxide (Librium). An initial dose of 50 mg is given by mouth. This dosage can be repeated after 1 hour if the patient remains extremely agitated. Around-the-clock dosage of chlordiazepoxide is usually scheduled over the next 4–5 days.

At the Westchester County Medical Center, we use the following procedure:

50 mg of chlordiazepoxide every 6 hours P.O. × four doses, followed by
25 mg q.i.d. P.O. × eight doses, followed by
10 mg q.i.d. P.O. × eight doses.

An order is also written for chlordiazepoxide 50 mg by mouth every 6 hours p.r.n. for any signs of withdrawal, such as tachycardia greater than 100/min, temperature greater than 38.3°C, hypertension with systolic pressure greater than 160 and diastolic pressure greater than 100, and nausea and vomiting. The medication should be held and the patient reevaluated if at any time he or she is not easily arousable, has slurred speech or nystagmus, or if ataxia appears (Kierzenbaum, personal communication, 1991). A rare but potentially lethal complication is oversedation, aspiration, or both. In uncomplicated alcohol withdrawal, although I.V. hydration may be given, the patient often can take medication by mouth. Occasionally, if a patient is uncooperative, initial doses of chlordiazepoxide are given i.m. Sometimes, because of marked confusion due to delirium or due to medical/surgical necessity, the patient takes nothing by mouth and receives chlordiazepoxide I.V. The procedure (Robert Vigdor, personal communication, 1991) would then be:

50 mg of chlordiazepoxide I.V. drip for 4 hours up to four times
Monitor the vital signs
Then, 25 mg I.V. drip over 6 hours for a 24-hour period
Repeat the last step another 24 hours if necessary
Patient should always be easily arousable.

Manufacturers' instructions for I.V. preparations should be followed. The chlordiazepoxide solution can irritate veins. For this reason, the use of lorazepam may be preferred with appropriate dosage (Kierzenbaum, personal communication, 1991).

Alcohol is cross-tolerant with all the benzodiazepines and most sedatives, such as the barbiturates. Therefore, the administration of such substances may suppress expected alcohol withdrawal signs and symptoms.

STANDARD GUIDELINES OR PROTOCOL

A standard protocol or guidelines should govern the treatment of patients for alcohol detoxification, to prevent alcohol withdrawal syndrome, or both (see Table 7.1). Such a protocol usually advises administering the minimal but sufficient amount of benzodiazepine needed to take the average patient through alcohol withdrawal. For some patients, a higher dosage is necessary. In rare situations, the dosage must be reduced because the patient is over-sedated. Although oversedation is rare, aspiration is the primary serious potential complication of the treatment of alcohol withdrawal syndrome with benzodiazepine. This should not happen if the patient is observed closely and regularly and if the dosage of the benzodiazepine is withheld for a patient who is not easily arousable.

If the patient does not respond to the standard protocol or guidelines, an etiology other than alcohol withdrawal syndrome is to be suspected. It would be a mistake to repeat the protocol if it was properly administered the first time. If there is no significant improvement in the alcohol withdrawal syndrome, an aggressive work-up must be done to find an etiology of the clinical picture. Infection, including HIV infection, head injury, blood loss, shock, and cardiac and renal diseases, among other causes, are all to be considered.

The guidelines and protocol also include Mylanta and Milk of Magnesia for common gastrointestinal symptoms, Tylenol for headaches, and thiamine and multivitamins for vitamin deficiencies that can cause other complications.

Table 7.1. Guidelines for Alcohol Detoxification Admission Orders[a]

		If no plate, print patient's name, chart no., and sex	
			PHYSICIAN ORDER SHEET
DATE	TIME	DIAGNOSIS	Noted by Sig./Title/Hr.

ALLERGIES:
Admit to Detoxification Unit
Bed rest as needed; Diet:
Vital signs q.i.d. for 5 days; CBC, urinalysis
Urine for toxicology; VDRL; SMAC; PT
HBs Ag (hepatitis surface antigen)
X-ray chest PA, EKG (for patients aged 40 and over)
Multivitamins 1 tablet b.i.d. P.O.
Thiamine 100 mg t.i.d. P.O.
Librium 50 mg P.O. q6h × 4 doses
Librium 25 mg P.O. q.i.d. × 8 doses to follow 50 mg
  series
Librium 10 mg P.O. q.i.d. × 8 doses to follow 25 mg
  series
Librium 50 mg P.O. q6h p.r.n. for any signs of withdrawal
  (tachycardia, hypertension, tremulousness)
Mylanta 45 cc P.O. q6h for indigestion p.r.n.
Milk of Magnesia 45 cc P.O. qhs p.r.n. for constipation
Tylenol tablets 650 mg P.O. q4h p.r.n. for headache
WITHHOLD LIBRIUM AND CALL PHYSICIAN IF
  PATIENT IS NOT EASILY AROUSABLE

PHYSICIAN'S SIGNATURE: M.D.
(DEA #1)

[a] Adapted from Alcoholism Treatment Services, Westchester County Medical Center.

USE OF LORAZEPAM IN THE TREATMENT OF ALCOHOL WITHDRAWAL

It is possible, theoretically, to substitute equivalent doses of lorazepam for chlordiazepoxide. This substitution seems especially appropriate for patients with severe liver disease because the lorazepam has a simpler and more predictable metabolic pathway and its accumulation in the plasma is insignificant (14). Such processes are related to the glucuoronidation in the kidney and other organs before excretion in the urine. Therefore, the body's ability to excrete lorazepam is not affected by hepatitis or cirrhosis (Kierzenbaum, personal communication, 1991). Our alcohol detoxification unit finds lorazepam to be less effective than chlordiazepoxide for the treatment and prevention of alcohol withdrawal syndrome because lorazepam increases sedation and allows only marginal control of autonomic excitation

(Vigdor, personal communication, 1991). Whenever possible, we favor chlordiazepoxide. With either agent, adjustment of dosage may be necessary because of a particular patient's needs.

USE OF PARALDEHYDE IN THE TREATMENT OF ALCOHOL WITHDRAWAL

Another technique that was popular 15 or 20 years ago and is still used at some centers for the treatment of alcohol withdrawal syndrome is paraldehyde (15). Pharmacologically, this substance is most similar to alcohol. Until the patient is asleep, 10 cc i.m. are given every hour. If the patient is more than 45 years old, 8 cc are commonly prescribed. Three doses are usually sufficient.

After the initial dose, the same amount of paraldehyde is given every 4 hours for 3 days. Continuing the dosage for more than 3 days can cause sterile abscesses, and patients who are stuporous from paraldehyde cannot be fed or made to cooperate. Vomiting and aspiration can be dangerous complications. After 3 days of sleep with appropriate hydration, the patient can be expected to have recovered from the alcohol withdrawal syndrome. It may be advisable to taper the frequency of paraldehyde during the last days, perhaps to every 8 hours. Patients who tolerate alcohol can take paraldehyde by mouth. Physical dependency on paraldehyde can develop if it is used for more than 10 days. Patients may need to be switched to a tranquilizer after 3 days on use. There is usually a distinct odor in the hospital unit from the breakdown products of paraldehyde that are eliminated through respiration.

USE OF ALCOHOL IN THE TREATMENT OF ALCOHOL WITHDRAWAL

Although we do not favor this approach, alcohol itself can be used as a possible treatment of alcohol withdrawal. In one study, 22 alcoholic burn patients received alcohol with I.V. infusion at the rate of 0.02–0.06 g/kg/ hour and achieved a low but measurable blood alcohol level (2–8 mg/dl) (16). This study reported no sedative or toxic effects and no appearance of withdrawal in alcoholic burn patients (16). We know of no systematic studies that have established the efficacy and safety of this approach, although we have heard word-of-mouth reports of this treatment or variations of it at a few other centers. The rationale is that, because most alcoholics return to alcohol consumption shortly after discharge, there is no reason to institute a withdrawal program.

With patients who have moderate-to-severe burn or trauma injuries, this approach would then require alcohol maintenance throughout several weeks of hospitalization that may include surgery. Even with patients who have a more abbreviated hospitalization, the maintenance of alcohol dependence seems a pessimistic and perhaps demeaning approach to patient care. In our opinion, the patient and family should be thoroughly informed by the medical/nursing team of the dangers of excessive alcohol intake.

As mentioned elsewhere, a burn or trauma injury is often experienced as a "brush with death." In the aftermath of the accident, a person may be able to consider making changes in his or her life that he or she could not previously make. Withdrawing the patient from alcohol as part of the treatment allows the patient to begin this process. As we describe below, additional support is usually necessary to pursue these changes.

Wernicke-Korsakoff Syndrome

Two rare alcohol conditions can occur individually or in combination in alcoholics who are nutritionally deprived. The conditions demonstrate specific damage to the brain and central nervous system with profound mental changes (10). The first condition, Korsakoff's psychosis, also referred to as *confabulatory psychosis*, is characterized by impaired memory in an otherwise alert and mentally intact individual. Memory impairment develops gradually and the patient usually has limited understanding of the memory loss. The patient frequently makes up responses (*confabulations*) in attempts to cover up blatant memory gaps. The patient can recover partially or completely with treatment.

The second condition, Wernicke's encephalopathy, appears suddenly and is characterized by ophthalmoplegia and ataxia followed by mental changes. The patient tends to be somnolent, confused, slow to reply, and has a characteristic ocular disturbance—paresis or paralysis of the external recti, nystagmus, and a disturbance of conjugate gaze. Proper treatment usually brings improvement in the ocular palsies within hours and improvement is complete within several days. The global confusional state is also reversible.

Both of these conditions are medical emergencies. The treatment is an initial 50 mg of thiamine (vitamin B1) I.V., followed by 50 mg i.m. daily until normal diet is resumed. Subsequent oral thiamine, 100 mg three times a day, should be given. Parenteral feeding and the administration of vitamin B complex is necessary if the patient is unable to eat. Other associated conditions, such as heart failure, must be treated. Behavioral problems must be treated symptomatically as well.

Prolonged Delirium in Alcoholics

Alcoholics admitted to our burn unit frequently develop a sustained delirium starting on the second, third, or fourth day and lasting 1–2 weeks or even longer. This occurs despite vigorous treatment for alcohol withdrawal along with excellent burn and medical management.

The clinical picture is similar to that of the burn delirium frequently seen in patients who has burns over more than 25% of their body surface, but this sustained delirium also appears to occur with much smaller burns in the alcoholic. Some patients have a confabulatory picture resembling Korsakoff's psychosis, but the patients are not characteristically alert. However, medication for pain may be influencing this presentation. Sometimes, the delirium of patients whose pain medication is tapered will improve. The prognosis is good for return to previous mental functioning after the patient has recovered physically. As described elsewhere in this book, the use of antipsychotic medications should be considered for patients with prolonged delirium and psychotic manifestations.

Recognition and Treatment of Chronic Alcoholism

A common tragedy in modern medicine occurs if a trauma or burn victim's life is saved through state-of-the-art critical care, and the person subsequently dies from complications of alcoholism that was present at the time of the accident but remained untreated.

After the patient passes through the acute phase of treatment for the burn and trauma and is medically and surgically stable, the treatment team usually shifts their attention to rehabilitation, sometimes forgetting the issues of alcohol withdrawal faced earlier in the hospitalization. Physician contact with a patient may be minimal as the patient moves toward discharge and perhaps outpatient follow-up. A window of opportunity for addressing the issues of alcohol abuse may be overlooked.

Even if patients have been through an alcohol withdrawal treatment phase, they usually forget this aspect of treatment as soon as they become alcohol-free in the hospital. At this point, the patient almost certainly will minimize his or her alcoholic background. However, after the patient stabilizes medically, the entire treatment team *must* evaluate and diagnose the presence of an alcohol problem and move forward to confront the patient with this problem constructively.

Alcohol withdrawal syndrome treatment during the acute phase of hospitalization is conclusive evidence of alcoholism. The presence of an enlarged liver or abnormal liver function tests confirm this fact and are useful in subsequent discussions with the patient. The family often provides a clear history of alcohol problems that the patient may minimize or deny.

Some patients remind everyone that they are alcoholic by their demanding to leave the hospital and openly expressing desires to "have a drink." Other patients show a pleasant demeanor that may not suggest underlying alcoholism.

Even if the diagnosis is unapparent, every patient should be clinically screened for the diagnosis of alcoholism. A simple way of doing this is to pose the CAGE questions (17). Two or more affirmative answers to the questions are generally indicative of alcoholism, and any positive response should raise a high suspicion of alcoholism and merit further investigation.

CAGE QUESTIONS
1. Have you ever felt the need to CUT down your drinking?
2. Have you ever felt ANNOYED by criticism about your drinking?
3. Have you had GUILTY feelings about your drinking?
4. Have you ever taken a morning "EYE opener"? (17)

Cloniger suggests that there are at least two kinds of alcoholics (18). Although they are not necessarily discrete disease entities, understanding these two kinds may make diagnosis easier. The type 1 alcoholic does not usually start ingesting alcohol until after age 25. This person can lose control when drinking and easily becomes psychologically dependent. Type 2 starts drinking at an earlier age and is much more likely to get into fights and trouble with the law while drinking. Type 2 rarely has guilt or fears about alcohol dependence. Women are more likely to be type 1 and there are mixtures of both types in both men and women (see Table 7.2).

The patient who has been hospitalized for a burn or trauma injury usually develops an emotional attachment to the surgeon and to the burn/trauma team that saved his or her life. Mostly, these are positive feelings with an underlying transferential meaning relating to earlier nurturing relationships. For this reason, with many patients, the surgeon and the burn/trauma team can constructively confront the patient about his or her drinking problem. This type of discussion may have more potential value in the hospital, after the patient stabilizes, than during the casual outpatient medical visit when the physician delivers admonitions about drinking. The surgeon, in particular, can convey his or her own wish that the life-saving efforts just performed should not be in vain. The surgeon should review directly with the

Table 7.2 Kind of Alcoholism[a]

Characteristic Features	Kind of Alcoholism	
	Type 1	Type 2
Usual age of onset (yr)	After 25	Before 25
Spontaneous alcohol-seeking behavior (inability to abstain)	Infrequent	Frequent
Fighting and arrests (when drinking)	Infrequent	Infrequent
Psychological dependence (loss of control)	Infrequent	Infrequent
Guilt and fear about alcohol dependence	Frequent	Infrequent
Personality traits		
Novelty seeking	Low	High
Harm avoidance	High	Low
Reward dependence	High	Low

[a] Adapted from Cloniger CR. Neurogenic adaptive mechanisms in alcoholism. Science 1987;236:410–415.

patient the poor prognosis of an individual who has had an alcohol withdrawal syndrome or who has abnormal liver function tests.

It may be inappropriate to be confrontational if the patient has a residual organic mental syndrome, severe depression, or residual symptoms of posttraumatic stress disorder. However, when the patient is psychologically intact and medically stable, we do not hesitate to confront him or her with the seriousness of the alcohol problem. We tell the patient our concern or even share our sadness that he or she has a poor prognosis because of the untreated alcohol problem.

The psychiatrist and other members of the psychosocial team should be certain that if the patient has a dual diagnosis (with affective disorder or schizophrenia as the most common second diagnosis), a clear follow-up treatment plan is developed recognizing the underlying alcoholism.

It becomes the task of the surgical, nursing, and psychosocial teams to encourage the patient to accept a referral to Alcoholics Anonymous (AA); to another reputable, available rehabilitation program; or to both. The family must be involved and interviewed by a member of the psychosocial team. Often, family members themselves are alcoholics who have facilitated the alcohol problem in the primary patient. Referral of the family members, especially spouse and children, can help the hospitalized patient get help. Even if the patient will not accept help, other family members may benefit from such groups.

We often encourage the alcoholic patient to request that a member of AA visit him during hospitalization. At our institution, an AA member visits only if the patient personally makes the request. Although anyone can go to an AA group, such groups tend to take on the socioeconomic characteristics of the area where they meet. Some groups primarily include executives and professionals; others may be mainly blue collar workers. Some groups have a successful mixture. The psychosocial team should be aware of the characteristics of the groups so that the best possible match can be made (9).

It is rare for an alcoholic to achieve abstinence without outside assistance. Simply to detoxify the patient and only to treat the trauma/burn injury is an unworkable, superficial approach. We have discussed above the meaning of a brush with death and how this may spur a person to make changes that might not have been made otherwise. Even if the patient is motivated for such change, we find that a referral for psychological follow-up, including but not necessarily limited to AA, is definitely necessary.

CASE STUDY

Ms. M., a 54-year-old single legal secretary, was admitted with a burn over 20% of her body. She had fallen asleep with a lighted cigarette in her hand and her nightgown had caught fire. The patient admitted that she had probably had too much to drink that night but denied any significant history of alcohol abuse. A blood alcohol level was not taken on admission because the doctor felt that a woman with such a responsible job would not have a drinking problem.

The patient's resuscitation was complicated by alcohol withdrawal and a prolonged period of confusion. At times she carried on a coherent and obviously intelligent conversation; at other times she was hardly aware of her surroundings and suffered severe memory deficits. After a thorough evaluation by psychiatry and a work-up suggested by neurology, it was decided that she had significant brain changes (Wernicke's) resulting from years of alcohol abuse. Her family confirmed she had a long history of depression and alcohol abuse and was no longer allowed to drive because of two DWI convictions.

Near the end of Ms. M.'s hospital stay, when her burns were healed and her mental status had cleared somewhat, the psychiatrist and psychiatric clinical nurse specialist met once again with her. Ms. M. enjoyed a positive relationship with them because they had seen her regularly throughout her hospitalization. The mental health team assured her that she would recover from the injuries, but that unfortunately she had a grave prognosis. They talked about the damage to her brain caused by alcohol and expressed their concern that if she went home without further alcohol rehabilitation she would likely be dead in a short time.

Ms. M. accepted an inpatient alcohol treatment program and was eventually able to return to work. The long-term outcome is yet unknown.

The importance of this case is that it shows that the psychiatric team has the responsibility to encourage alcohol treatment and is in a good position to push for that goal when it has established a good rapport with the patient.

Barbiturate and Benzodiazepine Dependency

Patients who take high doses of sedatives, such as barbiturates or benzodiazepines, either prescribed by a physician or in situations of abuse may have become physically dependent on them. Such patients may, on occasion, present to the emergency room with a burn or a trauma injury. Most are not in severe withdrawal when they are seen, but require treatment within 24 hours. Because patients who abuse substances often do not give accurate histories, their conditions may not be initially recognized. A patient may also be in a coma and, thus, be unable to give a history. A toxic screen from urine or blood can be helpful in these situations, but the results are frequently unavailable in the first 24 hours. Problems of overdose require immediate treatment in the emergency room.

The clinical signs and symptoms of withdrawal from potent sedative barbiturates with a short-to-intermediate half-life can occur in users taking as little as 800 mg/day for 6 weeks (19). If benzodiazepine is the drug abused, mild-to-moderate withdrawal is commonly seen in individuals taking two to three times the usual clinical dosage over a several-month period (20). When benzodiazepines have been used a month or more, withdrawal symptoms are possible even if the patient took only the usual clinical dosage. Mild withdrawal symptoms are evident even when the patient has only used the drug for a few weeks.

Early symptoms of withdrawal, which are those seen in the first 24–48 hours, are apprehension, dysphoria, intolerance to bright lights and noises, hypotension, anorexia, hyperreflexia, muscle weakness, and muscle twitches. Tremor tends to be coarse, rhythmic, nonpatterned, evident during voluntary movement, and subsiding at rest.

Seizures can begin on the second or third day and last as long as 8 days. They can progress to status epilepticus with hyperpyrexia and cardiovascular collapse.

From the third to the eighth day, and lasting as long as 3–14 days, a delirium tremens-like syndrome may develop, possibly with marked confusion and a severe panic state. Hallucinations, psychotic manifestations, and a delirium indistinguishable from alcoholic withdrawal and delirium tremens can occur. The intensity of these symptoms disappears over 3–14 days, although anxiety, sleep disturbances, and autonomic nervous system irregularities may continue in mild form for up to 6 months (19, 21, 22). Drugs given to treat the acute burn and trauma condition may mask this clinical picture. Narcotics are not cross-tolerant to alcohol, benzodiazepines, and barbiturates, but the last three are cross-tolerant to each other. After benzodiazepine withdrawal is recognized, it is usually relatively simple to avoid the serious consequences of withdrawal by gradual reduction of the dose.

Barbiturate withdrawal can be the most difficult drug withdrawal syndrome to treat and can produce the most severe extremes of the clinical picture described above. The administration of a short-acting barbiturate to treat barbiturate withdrawal is tricky; the lethal dosage is not much greater in chronic use than it is in neophyte use.

One method to determine the amount of barbiturate needed to treat withdrawal is the pentobarbital test dose method (23). According to this method, after waiting a few hours to ascertain that no drug has been taken recently, the patient is given 200 mg pentobarbital. One hour after the test dosage, the patient is evaluated for the presence of intoxication (expected if the patient is intolerant). If the patient appears intoxicated and has marked drowsiness, dysarthria, coarse lateral nystagmus, positive Romberg tests, and a loss of fine motor coordination, then only mild tolerance is involved and the risk of withdrawal reaction is low. If at the end of an hour the patient shows no signs of intoxication or withdrawal, the daily requirement to prevent withdrawal is estimated at between 400 and 600 mg/day.

If the patient shows signs of abstinence with tremors, muscle twitches, hyperpyrexia, and postural hypotension, marked tolerance and severe withdrawal are expected. Then the total daily dose required for the patient is likely to be 800–1600 mg/day of pentobarbital. The patient should be given 200–300 mg of an oral, short-acting barbiturate and reevaluated every 2 hours. When the patient becomes intoxicated, the entire amount of drug required over the next 24 hours should be calculated and then given in equally divided doses every 4–6 hours for approximately 2 days. The pentobarbital should then be decreased by 100 mg/day.

In instances of mild-to-moderate tolerance to barbiturates, we may substitute equivalent doses of a benzodiazepine such as lorazepam. This may avoid the overdose problems associated with pentobarbital (19). There are other techniques for diagnosing and following the progress of barbiturate withdrawal (19, 23). One approach consists of converting the approximate dosage of the sedative to a phenobarbital equivalent that has a half-life of 24 hours. Usually, 1 unit of sedative, such as pentobarbital or 300 mg of methaqualone or its equivalents, is equal to 30 mg of phenobarbital. The total dosage of phenobarbital is divided into four doses and given every 6 hours. After 2 days, it is gradually reduced to 30 mg/day. For emergency control of withdrawal symptoms, 100–200 mg i.m. can be given as needed.

If nothing can be given by mouth, an I.V. schedule is set up. For emergency surgery, the anesthesiologist must be informed of existing history and the progress achieved in withdrawing the patient and preventing a withdrawal syndrome. The time taken for withdrawal can be varied under emergency conditions. However, the possibility of seizures should always be considered if abrupt withdrawal is undertaken.

Narcotic Dependence

It is rare to see an immediate acute withdrawal from a narcotic in a burn or trauma patient. The narcotic given for pain management usually masks or prevents narcotic withdrawal. However, if the patient develops tolerance to the narcotic because of previous or current narcotic usage, a higher than average dosage of pain medication is required for adequate pain control.

A patient who was in a methadone program before admission may be continued on methadone during hospitalization, although an additional narcotic is necessary for pain control. The methadone program should be contacted to confirm the dosage and to arrange referral back to the program after discharge.

On rare occasions, if narcotics are not required for pain control, the patient may have narcotic withdrawal symptoms while in the hospital. These symptoms can be treated with methadone starting with an initial 10-mg dose. If the withdrawal symptoms persist, an additional 5–10 mg may be repeated every 4–6 hours. The total dosage in 24 hours equals the dose for the second day (seldom more than 40 mg/day). This is given in divided doses two or three times per day. The dosage is then decreased by 5 mg/day for heroin withdrawal. Methadone withdrawal may require a slower dose reduction. Pentazocine-dependent patients should be detoxified on pentazocine (24).

Cocaine does not require detoxification or withdrawal, but these patients can become depressed subsequently.

Clonidine, a short-acting non-narcotic that is an α_2-agonist, is to relieve nausea, vomiting, and diarrhea that are part of the opioid withdrawal syndrome. Clonidine, 0.1–0.2 mg, is given every 3 hours, not to exceed 0.8 mg/day. When stabilized, the dosage is tapered over 2 weeks. Hypotension can be a side effect (24).

If nausea and vomiting occur, they can be treated symptomatically with Compazine or Tigan. If the patient has a history of narcotic usage, he or she may verbalize a desire for extra pain medication while in the hospital and show a knowledge of the dosage and the various types of medication. The pain from burn and trauma is real and quite severe. The patient who has been dependent on narcotics often requires a higher dosage to achieve pain control because of tolerance. It is better to err on the high side to achieve adequate pain control.

The dosage of narcotics should be tapered during the recovery phase in the hospital. As we have noted elsewhere, adequate pain management will not turn anyone into a street addict. Similarly, addiction to a narcotic is not a reason to withhold adequate pain control.

Individuals who sustain a burn or a trauma injury may be abusing numerous other drugs. The clinical picture depends on the nature of the drug or drugs (mixed substance abuse is common) and on the effect of pain medication (usually narcotic) required for pain control. When there is doubt about the nature of the substance the patient has been taking, the approach should be supportive and conservative until toxicology tests reveal what the specific substances are (Kierzenbaum, personal communication, 1991). Mixed substance abuse with alcohol is very common. If alcohol is known or suspected to be one of the substances, the best approach is to focus first on alcohol withdrawal as the only physiologically dangerous syndrome (Vigdor, personal communication, 1991).

We have seen a few patients with flash burns that occurred during the free-basing of cocaine, or with flame injuries from a house fire in a "crack house." By the time that they reach the emergency room, the acute effects of the cocaine have already passed and the secondary lethargy and hypersomnia with apathy are not serious problems during the acute burn care. We expect a similar picture in patients taking stimulants such as amphetamines. However, as these patients stabilize, they may show marked depression with potential suicidal ideation. They should be watched closely for such symptoms.

Patients who have been using psychedelic drugs (LSD, PCP, TCH, marijuana, and others) at the time of a burn or trauma injury can present a clinical picture of acute psychosis that may be indistinguishable from acute schizophrenia. In these instances, substance abuse is more likely to include visual and tactile hallucinations and illusions. These patients are more likely to have dilated pupils. There may be a labile and inappropriate affect, as well as an organic mental syndrome with cognitive deficits. Such patients can also have a loss of motor coordination, spontaneous nystagmus, and hyperesthesias (19). If necessary, antipsychotic drugs such as haloperidol (Haldol), chlorpromazine (Thorazine), or others can symptomatically treat these psychotic manifestations. However, the acute effects of these substances are usually over within several hours. Flashbacks of drug experiences may occur and sometimes be indicative of underlying psychological problems.

Patients who have been inhaling glue and solvents rarely have persistent psychiatric symptoms on presentation. But these patients can have serious medical problems such as hepatitis with liver failure, kidney failure, decreased pulmonary function, peripheral neuropathy, cardiac arrhythmias, and other complications (19).

Any patient who has used needles to inject him- or herself with substances is a candidate for HIV infection, which is discussed elsewhere in this book.

Problems in Managing the Drug Abuser in the Hospital

Patients who are substance abusers may present special problems in management. Their knowledge of narcotics and other drugs can lead them to demand more pain medication. As mentioned, because of tolerance, they may actually require a higher dosage for pain control. If possible, it can be especially useful to switch the patient to long-acting morphine, as outlined in a pain protocol in Chapter 1. This approach minimizes the clock watching and patient interaction with the staff about pain medication. As described, the dosage needs to be tapered before discharge.

If it is suspected that the patient is receiving illicit drugs in the hospital, daily urine tests should be given. Medication should be given to such patients under direct observation to prevent them from saving the medication and using it later in increased dosages.

Patients who are substance abusers often have antisocial personalities. They tend to be easily frustrated; to be ambivalent in interpersonal relationships, demanding, and unable to plan ahead; to desire immediate gratification of whatever need is foremost, be concerned about what other people are going to do for them, and constantly test the rules (19).

Caring for such patients can lead to significant management problems in the burn and trauma setting. The staff must be consistent and clearly spell out what is expected of the patient. The patient's behavior may be quite provocative and cause the busy, hard-working staff to react with anger. In some situations, the patient's behavior reflects great insecurity and immaturity in his or her reaction to staff support and care—which may be the types of attention that he or she has never experienced before. The patient's antisocial behavior is usually a basic part of his or her personality and will not often be mitigated by the most empathic and well-meaning staff. Regular input from the psychosocial team can be particularly helpful for these patients. Manipulative and acting out behavior can be picked up early and consistent treatment plans developed.

CASE STUDY

Mr. G. was a 29-year-old involved in a high-speed motor vehicle accident that resulted in the death of a 28-year-old mother and her 4-year-old child. The patient had a blood alcohol level indicating intoxication and, in addition, had a long history of drug addiction. His injuries included bilateral compound fractures of both lower extremities, six broken ribs, and several facial lacerations. He required an early trip to the operating room for a ruptured spleen. Ten days after admission, Mr. G. required a below-the-knee amputation of his left leg. Although he was monitored closely, he showed no evidence of alcohol or drug withdrawal after hospitalization.

Staff reaction to Mr. G was thinly veiled anger. They cared for him but made frequent comments about the amount of medication that he required for pain. One nurse expressed the feelings of many when she was heard to say, "For what he did, he should suffer." In this situation, the mental health team was needed for patient, family, *and* staff. Although Mr. G. was initially belligerent and demanding, after a psychiatrist started working with him and his feelings of remorse, guilt, and grief, his attitude toward the staff improved significantly. However, his need for pain medications was an ongoing problem and the nurses complained that he could not possibly be in so much pain. They expressed fear that they were supporting his drug habit and that the amount of narcotics he received could kill him. The psychiatric clinical nurse specialist worked with the staff to communicate the patient's understandable tolerance to narcotics and higher requirements for pain medication. The staff discovered that when the patient's requirements for pain medication were adequately calculated, he was much easier to care for because he was able to cooperate.

In the final weeks of his hospitalization, and before his transfer to a drug rehabilitation setting, Mr. G. was being weaned off MS Contin and was on p.r.n. morphine elixir. Suddenly, the nurses again began to complain about his demands and said that he would never become a contributing member of society. When his pain medications were reviewed, it became immediately clear that the problem was not that Mr. G. had become suddenly demanding again, but that a new resident had lowered the morphine dosage too rapidly. Mr. G.

was suffering from a combination of physical withdrawal and poor pain management.

This case study illustrates how necessary the monitoring of various dynamics is in a trauma patient with a history of addictive behavior. Although the staff is usually skillful in managing pain issues, a new set of concerns and feelings emerges with these patients.

Of additional interest was Mr. G.'s younger sister (age 20), who visited him frequently at the hospital and agreed to seek help for her own alcohol problem. Although their parents maintained that neither child had a problem, they were able to utilize their son's injury as an opportunity to address their own estrangement from each other.

Many patients with substance abuse problems have a dual diagnosis. This means they also have an underlying psychiatric disorder. Alcohol, an abused substance, is commonly combined with other abused substances. Depression of one form or another, particularly with a major affective disorder, is found in at least half of all patients with substance abuse. Schizophrenia, anxiety disorders—including panic disorder—and other personality disorders including antisocial personality, dependent personality, and borderline personality—may also coexist with substance abuse.

Hospitalization for acute burn and trauma injury invariably brings about withdrawal from the abused substance and a drug-free period during the hospitalization. This period becomes valuable for the diagnosis of coexisting psychiatric conditions and an opportunity—a unique window—for the patient to develop some insight and understanding of the psychiatric condition that led to the substance abuse. An important role for the psychiatrist and psychosocial team is to work with the patient toward this understanding.

For example, a person may have taken a substance to ward off depression. Or the patient may have medicated him- or herself to handle disturbing thoughts or panic symptoms. More complex reasons for substance abuse may be related to uncontrolled and repressed impulses, ambivalent relationships, and conflicts only understood through a careful psychological evaluation of the patient in a drug-free state.

Hospitalization gives the staff an opportunity to institute antidepressive therapy, treatment for panic disorder, or antipsychotic medication for psychotic conditions. The therapeutic alliance that is established with the consultant or psychosocial team can continue in outpatient treatment or be helpful in making a referral.

Referrals should be made to outpatient programs, drug rehabilitation units, AA, NA (Narcotics Anonymous), and similar self-help groups. As mentioned earlier, it is particularly meaningful if patients become motivated to make their own phone calls regarding appointments for follow-up for the above programs and services.

It is easy to become discouraged in work with alcoholics and other substance abusers because of the low success rate in various treatment programs. However, we view every hospitalization as a critical opportunity to aid patient and family. Let us not, as caregivers, take on the pessimism and complacency that pervades an addict's life.

References

1. Lowenfels AB, Miller TT. Alcohol and trauma. Ann Emerg Med 1984;13:1056–1060.
2. Lindenbaum GA, Carroll SF, Daskal I, Kapusnick R. Patterns of alcohol and drug abuse in an urban trauma center. J Trauma 1985;29:1654–1658.
3. Thal ER, Bost RO, Anderson RJ. Effects of alcohol and other drugs on traumatized patients. Arch Surg 1985;120:708–712.
4. Bailey DN. Drug use in patients admitted to a university trauma center. J Anal Toxicol 1990;14:22–24.
5. Brodzka W, Thornhill HL, Howard S. Burns: causes and risk factors. Arch Phys Med Rehabil 1985;66:746–752.
6. Howland J, Hingson R. Alcohol as a risk factor for injuries or death due to fires and burn—Review of literature. Public Health Rep 1987;102:475–483.
7. Berry CC, Patterson JL, Wachtel TL, Frank HA. Behavioral factors in burn mortality and length of stay in hospital. Burns 1984;10:409–414.
8. Tikellis JI, Spillert CR, Syval W, Lazaro EJ. Beneficial effects of ethanol on experimental burn. Am Surg 1986;52:53–55.
9. Ewing JA. Substance abuse: alcohol. In: Houpt JL, Brodie HKH, eds. Psychiatry. vol 3. Consultation-liaison psychiatry and behavioral medicine. Philadelphia: JB Lippincott Company, 1986:113–126.
10. Hackett IP. Alcoholism: acute and chronic states. In: Hackett IP, Cassem NH, eds. Massachusetts General Hospital handbook of general psychiatry. St. Louis: CV Mosby, 1978.
11. Hayes SL, Pablo G, Radomski J, et al. Ethanol and oral diazepam absorption. N Engl J Med 1977;296:186–187.
12. Jones JD, Barber B, Engras L, Heimbach D. Alcohol use and burn injury. J Burn Care Rehab 1991;12:148–152.
13. Hoffman von Bendel J. Delirium tremens in accident surgery (in German). Aktuel Traumatol 1983;13:250–252.
14. Solomon J. Double-blind comparison of lorazepam and chlordiazepoxide in the treatment of the acute alcoholism abstinence syndrome. Clin Ther 1983;79–83.
15. Glickman LS. Psychiatric consultation in the general hospital. New York: Marcel Dekker Inc., 1980.
16. Hansbrough JF, Zapata-Sirvent RL, Carroll WJ, Johnson R, Saunders CE, Barton CA. Administration of intravenous alcohol for prevention of withdrawal in alcoholic burn patients. Am J Surg 1984;148:266–269.
17. Bernadt MW, Mumford T, Taylor C, et al. Comparison of questionnaires and laboratory tests in detection of excessive drinking and alcohol. Lancet 1982;1:325.
18. Cloniger CR, Neurogenic adaptive mechanisms in alcoholism. Science 1987;236:410–415.
19. Ellinwood EH, Woody G, Krishnan RR. Treatment for drug abuse. In: Houpt JL, Brodie HKH, eds. Psychiatry. vol 3. Consultation-liaison psychiatry and behavioral medicine. Philadelphia: JB Lippincott Company, 1986:127–138.
20. Covi L, Lippmann HH, Pattison JH, et al. Length of treatment with anxiolytic sedation and response to their sudden withdrawal. Acta Psychiatr Scand 1973;49:51–64. Philadelphia: JB Lippincott Company, 1986:127–139.

21. Wikler A: Diagnosis and treatment of drug dependence of the barbiturate type. Am J Psychiatry 1968;125:759–765.
22. Kaplan H, Saddock BJ. Pocket handbook of clinical psychiatry. Baltimore: Williams & Wilkins, 1990:36–47.
23. Smith DE, Wesson DR. Phenobarbital technique for treatment of barbiturate dependence. Arch Gen Psychiatry 1971;15:56–60.
24. Greenspan L, Bakalar JB. Drug dependence: nonnarcotic agents. In: Kaplan H, Saddock BJ, eds. Comprehensive textbook of psychiatry. 4th ed. Baltimore: Williams & Wilkins, 1985:1003–1016.

Amputation and Replantation

Amputation

Amputation is the loss of a limb or body part because of a traumatic event, violence, an accident, or a medically necessitated event such as the removal of a diseased or infected part to preserve the life or health of the amputee. Whatever the cause, amputation represents a unique assault on the integrity and wholeness of the body, and a permanent loss. It causes an irreversible change in the person's body image. The many psychological and social consequences of the amputation are as important to the patient's healing as is the physical healing of the stump itself.

With the existence of microvascular surgery and other advancements of medical science, a discussion of amputation must address the psychological implications of replantation. No longer does the trauma automatically end with an amputation. An increasing number of fingers, toes, hands, arms, and legs are being reattached and made functional through a series of operations.

CHARACTERISTICS OF AMPUTEES

The most common causes of traumatic amputation are industrial accidents, which account for about 35% of the losses. Vehicular and domestic accidents account approximately for another 30% and 25%, respectively. The remainder of traumatic amputations fall into the categories of gunshot wounds, electrical injuries, and other causes (1). Not included in these statistics are amputations necessitated by disease processes and complications of illnesses such as diabetes, vascular compromise, and malignant tumors. While the sudden loss of limb carries the burden of lack of preparation, all amputations require the individual to make immense psychological and physical adjustments.

Although any person may fall victim to a sudden amputation, the statistics on amputation are similar to those on spinal cord injury: those injured are predominantly adolescents and young adults, and they are male more often than female (2). As with other accidents, victims of amputation tend to have a higher incidence of pre-injury psychological problems, a greater number of stressors in the year preceding the accident, and a greater incidence of alcohol and other substance abuse than the nonaccident population (3, 4).

Malec, in a study on personality factors associated with severe trauma disability (5), found that the sample population divided into three groups, with differing outcomes at long-term follow-up. Group 1 had an active role in their injuries, were more daring, and had less cautious attitudes. They were the better adjusted. Group 2 had a more passive, indirect role in their injuries (such as being passengers caught in auto accidents) and were less well adjusted. Group 3 were innocent victims of accidental happenings. These individuals showed the least adjustment. The findings suggest that the "very traits that predispose certain persons to serious injury may make then more resistant to stress and more active and energetic in coping" (6).

The problems of managing the amputee in the hospital, providing for rehabilitation, and assuring reentry into family and community remain difficult. Alteration of the body must be accommodated cognitively in the body concept and affectively in body esteem (6).

PHANTOM PHENOMENA

Phantom phenomena is where the patient experiences the amputated limb as still existing. It is a universal consequence of amputation. Phantom phenomena have been of great interest for many years to physicians, who wish to relieve their patients of the pain and mental difficulties caused thereby, and to researchers, who are still baffled by their precise etiology. Researchers often use different terminology for similar phenomena.

Ribbers et al. (7) make some helpful distinctions: *phantom phenomena* is the continuous awareness of a nonexisting (amputated) body part with a specific form, weight, or range of motion. *Phantom sensations*, then, are nonpainful sensations of the phantom limb. *Phantom pain* is the painful sensation felt in the stump or phantom limb that is due to neuroma, postoperative pain, and pain felt by abnormal sensitivity.

Phantom limb, as simple awareness, is thus more general than either phantom sensation or phantom pain, which are further distinguished by being nonpainful and painful awareness, respectively (7). This is an important distinction. While all amputees experience phantom sensation, a majority (more than 80%) experience phantom pain (8). At least one study found phantom pain in 100% of those studied (9).

ETIOLOGY OF PHANTOM PAIN

Theories explaining phantom phenomena fall into either organic or psychological categories, and organic theories include two subsets—peripheral and central.

Organic Theories of Phantom Phenomena

According to the peripheral theory of phantom phenomena, phantom limb sensations and pain are caused by nerve endings in the stump that continue to propagate impulses carried to the central nervous system. The brain designates these impulses as coming from the part of the body formerly innervated by the severed nerves; the impulses are perceived to come from the now amputated limb (10).

Most research supports peripheral theory, but the theory is incomplete. For example, electrical stimulation of the stump increases phantom sensation although local anesthesia abolishes phantom pain, at least while the anesthetic effects last (10). Also, although pathology in the stump such as scar tissue, bone fragments, stitch abscesses, and neuroma formation precipitate pain, such pain may continue even *after* healing. Peripheral theory also fails to explain why phantom pain does not follow the distribution of the severed nerves and why it occurs less often in amputees who are less than 6 years of age. As expected, central theories use central nervous system mechanisms to explain phantom phenomena. Sensations vary according to the level of the central nervous system considered most crucial, for example, spinal cord, reticular activating system of the brainstem, or cortical influence. Although contributing much to the understanding of phantom pain, no central theory argument satisfactorily explains how patients distinguish between phantom sensation and phantom pain. Some attribute phantom limb pain to spinal factors—mostly abnormal firing in the dorsal horns of the spinal cord. On reaching the brain, the circuits are experienced as painful. If the sensations are too strong, lasting, or painful, conscious inhibition is ineffective.

Emotional and psychological factors can also modulate the sensations experienced by the patient, by their input via autonomic paths that originate centrally. No effect is produced by surgically removing the peripheral source after these circuits are in operation. The fact that paraplegics (who have lost more peripheral input than amputees) experience phantom phenomena less often, less intensely, and more vaguely with respect to detail is used as an argument supporting higher central mechanisms as the determining factor (10).

Riddoch hypothesizes that a cortical representation of body image develops with time as a result of peripheral input from all of the senses (10). Amputation does not alter this body image, which becomes a fixed part of individual perception (11). Evidence for this cortical control theory includes the following three aspects: amputees can at times both produce sensations in and move the phantom limb voluntarily; phantom sensation of body parts that have greater cortical representation, such as fingers and toes, persist longer; and objects, such as rings and watches that have been worn so continuously that they have become part of the cortical representation, are often part of the phantom sensation. The gradual fading of the pain and lack of phantom sensations in patients with long-term anesthesia in the preamputated limb have been explained by a gradual reorganization of the central body image due to the changes in peripheral input before the amputation (11).

Psychological Theories of Phantom Phenomena

Psychological factors, by no means the sole cause of phantom phenomena, are widely recognized to contribute to the maintenance and amplification of phantom limb pain. Denial of the loss of a body part is the most commonly acknowledged psychological mechanism that plays a role in phantom limb pain. If pain is suppressed by conscious cortical paths, then this suppression may decrease because of unconscious needs to experience the pain. The pain is *real* as explained by the peripheral and central organic theories. Something that hurts is most certainly there. It hurts, and therefore it exists. The physical pain (because it is not suppressed) may be less painful than the psychological pain of having to face the reality of the loss of limb immediately.

In a study of amputees, Shulka et al. (12) reported phantom pains lasting longer in right-handed patients who lost the right hand than in those who lost their nondominant hands. Perhaps their pain of loss is greater due to a lost concept of the functional self. The right hand is used more by a right-hander and therefore gives more peripheral input.

Some suggest that phantom pain is a denial of the affect connected with the loss rather than a denial of the loss itself. Phantom pain has been compared to a dream that expresses unconscious wishes in a distorted and conflicted way. Phantom limbs often have gaps—they are not continuous and they often disappear in a telescoping manner. The patient feels that the limb is shriveling in size. Some see this shriveling as the expression of a conflict between the wish to hold on to the limb and the opposing wish to hold on to the reality (11).

The arguments against the role of denial in phantom pain are observations that phantom pain may last for decades even when the amputee has apparently accepted the loss well. No matter what the dynamics are, the majority of patients do report pain, and earlier research indicating phantom pain as being rare was probably influenced by patients who were afraid to talk about pain they thought must be in their minds (8).

Pain researchers now fairly uniformly document two main kinds of pain associated with amputations: rare intense pain, usually associated with environmental factors such as cold or humid weather or stress, or continuous background pain unrelated to environmental factors (7).

Regardless of the origin of the pain associated with an amputation, the pain requires intervention. Postoperative pain medications should be used liberally, and psychological stages of adjustment must be addressed. Patients need information to validate the legitimacy of their sensations and they need assurance that they are not going crazy or hallucinating. They must learn that their pain will likely decrease and that the staff will attend to the pain. Families also need careful explanations of the phenomena of phantom sensations and pain so that they can be supportive.

AMPUTATION AND THE GRIEF RESPONSE

Following an initial stage of shocked disbelief, amputees undergo intense grief similar to the experience of losing a loved, valued, and highly cathected object. This phase is similar to the acute state of mourning described in the previous chapter on psychological reactions. The patient mourns not only the limb, but also his or her former self-image.

Amputation is a profound assault on one's basic body image, around which the sense of self is organized. The body feels distorted and, therefore, the self feels distorted. The amputation may take on an unconscious meaning related to symbolic castration and, thus, may bring forth castration anxiety. The amputation may also be interpreted by the patient as a punishment. Indeed, in primitive cultures, amputation used to be, and still is today a punishment for crimes.

After an initial period of denial, the amputee usually enters a period of anger. Because one cannot be angry at something that does not exist, anger is likely to be displaced. (Displacement of anger is discussed further in the chapter on psychological reactions.) One may view anger as an important step toward mastering the shock and disbelief brought about by amputation.

Eventually, patients move through the early grief response and anticipate the next stage. From the psychodynamic perspective of a physician who has had an amputation, Stoudemire reports that he saw his prosthesis as a "bizarre, alien contraption, that initially I perceived as disappointing and repulsive . . . as not-self" (13). He goes on to acknowledge that accepting the prosthesis is a process of decathecting the old limb and recathecting the new limb even though it is inferior in all respects. The opportunity to obtain a prosthesis is often anticipated with unrealistic expectations that are likely to lead to initial disappointments for the patient and family. The artificial limb is lifeless and far from functional in the beginning (14).

The emotional isolation of an amputee has been seen as part of a vicious circle that can further hinder reintegration. People often avoid patients with a deformity because it reminds them of their own vulnerability and possible castration, mutilation, and losses. Even after a patient may have come to grips with his or her own loss, the difficulty others have with that loss can lead to more angry resentment in the patient and can serve to drive supports away. The support of other amputees, which is often found on rehabilitation units, can be invaluable at this time for the patient as well as struggling family and friends.

AMPUTATION AND FLASHBACK PHENOMENA

Flashbacks are the visual, tactile, and auditory components of the original accident that are experienced when the patient is awake. Flashbacks produce an anxiety response. They are usually vivid, recurring recollections of the injury. Also, the majority of amputees' nightmares show preoccupation with further injuries or anticipated incapacities resulting from the injury (15).

Specific kinds of flashbacks or combinations of them may be prognostic indicators of rehabilitation (16). Although the studies that are the basis for differentiating kinds of flashbacks were conducted with patients who had had hand amputations or hand injuries, their conclusions can probably be extended to all amputations.

The three kinds of flashbacks are:

1. *Replay.* A replaying of the events immediately preceding the accident and continuing until the time of injury.
2. *Appraisal.* An image of the injured hand immediately after replay.

3. *Projected.* An image of injuries worse than the real injury.

Regardless of injury type, patients with replay flashbacks were the most likely to return to their former employment (95.2%), and those with a combination of appraisal and projected were the least likely (10.3%) (16).

With an appraisal/projected combination flashback, the patient not only reexperiences the injury but also sees (projects) an injury worse than that which occurred. He or she therefore perceives little control over the injury process, is afraid of further injury, and avoids stimuli associated with the original injury. The more realistic replay flashbacks appear to serve a more positive purpose. Through them, patients can learn to master the event and thereby decrease their anxiety. They can also imagine ways that the outcome could have been different and perhaps come to feel that they can guard against future injury.

Patients with replay/projected combinations (55%) were divided approximately equally between a positive and a negative response to this replay of events up to, and including an exaggerated image of, the injury. By seeing that they could have sustained a more serious injury, they felt lucky to have escaped a worse one, and thus felt in control. But they also felt that circumstances beyond their control had kept them from experiencing a more severe injury and these feelings increased their anxiety and avoidance. In brief, the degree of control that a patient perceives he or she has over potential injury is a determining factor in his or her rehabilitation. How he or she arrives at this control may vary; the replay/projected combination can produce either a positive or a negative reaction to the perceived exaggerated image.

Patients with amputations should be encouraged to view nightmares and flashbacks as positive aspects of their emotional adjustment and to talk about their experiences in therapy. They can be encouraged to manage accompanying anxiety and startle reactions through relaxation and controlled breathing (15). Other times, psychotropic medications may be helpful.

AMPUTATIONS IN GERIATRIC PATIENTS

Most early studies of amputees did not include patients more than 70 years old; the mean age of patients in these studies was around 50 years. A more specific study by Frank et al. looked at amputations in older populations (17). His study divided subjects into two groups: one with a mean age of 47, another with a mean age of 75. The older amputees showed less depression and fewer psychological symptoms than the younger group, whose depression and symptoms after the amputation increased with time.

Significant evidence suggests that older amputees cope more effectively with amputation immediately following amputation and also as time passes. Perhaps many older patients have already accepted various changes in physical appearance and bodily capacity as well as losses of friends and loved ones. All loss is a kind of mini-death or foreshadowing of the ultimate loss of life. Older patients have an increased likelihood of having dealt with such situations. They have been "inoculated" with smaller doses of loss and have developed a sort of psychological immune system to loss in general. But older patients frequently have fewer social supports and decreased motivational factors for adaptation to prosthetic devices.

The loss of a limb in this population can be a final blow that leads them to resignation and, ultimately, to give up on life. Regardless of the age of the amputee, the outcome depends on the significance of the loss to that individual as well as on his or her personal coping skills.

AMPUTATIONS IN CHILDREN

Denial, a common defense among amputees, is not as rigid in children. Because an opportunity was given them to share loneliness and loss, all patients in a study of nine children aged 4–15 years quickly passed through the stage of denial (18). Some children are more insistent about knowing the truth than the adults around them.

CASE STUDY

A 6-year-old boy became angry with the nurses when they were reluctant to let him see his amputated leg during a dressing change. The nurses were afraid of seeing the shock on his face. The boy did not want his amputated leg covered with blankets. He wisely observed, "It is easier to get used to if I can see it."

Older children may develop unrealistic fantasies of recovery or cure. When she heard about the possibility of a prosthesis, one girl we followed remarked, "I hope I will have my artificial leg by summer so I can ride my bike."

Between the ages of 1 and 3 years, children establish a certain mental representation of their bodies as separate from the rest of the world. Amputation disturbs this concept of body image, which is closely linked to self-esteem. Although feelings are not often directly expressed by children, they may be exhibited through anxiety, depression, and confusion. Integration of a new self depends largely on the reactions of parents and others in the child's environment.

Family reactions depend on how the family has functioned in the past, the nature of the accident that caused the child's amputation, the child's age and response, and the way the team handles the situation. Psychological intervention with the family to help handle issues of guilt and self-blame are essential. The child is also likely to have feelings of guilt. Anger toward the child, although frequently denied, needs to be acknowledged as it is identified.

Family members show stages similar to the child's in the process of loss and mourning. Often, if the child is unable to move on to the next stage in the grieving process, there is at least some collusion, if not outright support, from the family for the fixation (18). Sometimes, family members project fears and conflicts onto the child when the child is ready to share his feelings with them. The child may assume the role of comforter as did a 4-year-old who patted his mother's arm and said, "Don't worry, Mom. I will be able to learn to walk with a wooden leg, just you wait and see."

Telling their child that there is no other choice and that they, as parents, must give consent to an amputation is, according to parents, one of the most painful experiences of their lives. Although they agree that their child needs to hear this information from them, most parents find the experience too painful and ask the doctor or mental health member of the team to initiate the communication. The more the parents can recognize and work through their own feelings of loss and resulting sadness and anger, the better they will handle the child's feelings and emotional needs. The time spent by the staff with parents is, in reality, also time spent with the child. For a further discussion on handling family reactions and the treatment team's reactions, see the chapters, "Care and Support of the Family" and "Care and Support of the Staff."

HAND AMPUTATIONS

Nearly 1 million Americans have a permanent loss of some portion of the hand or arm. Twenty-two percent of all industrial injuries during 1980 were hand injuries (15). How important is a hand? "We pursue our vocation and perhaps more importantly our avocation as bimanual creatures. We caress our loved ones with the hand, we greet a friend or acknowledge an individual with the right hand. Loss of these capabilities diminishes the individual" (19).

Amputations or deformities of the hand may have as much psychological impact on the patient, and consequently his family, as a deformity of the face. The hands are almost as emotionally expressive as the face and almost equally involved in communication and intimacy. The hands are more constantly in view than other limbs. The face is an essential expression of personality and emotionality; the hands are an expression of competence, skill, and tactile experiences. In addition to the changes in self-image, the great functional loss that comes with the loss of a hand creates extra psychological significance (15).

In a study of 67 patients with hand injuries, nightmares occurred following injury in 92% of the patients, flashbacks occurred in 88%, and affective lability occurred in 84%. These percentages are higher than the percentages of such reactions to other limb amputations (15).

PSYCHOLOGICAL INTERVENTIONS

The role of the mental health team seems obvious in the population of amputees. Management of phantom phenomena, assurance of a healthy resolution to loss, aid in reorganization of body image, and facilitation of a positive reintegration into life are all tasks enhanced by the involvement of well-trained, professional psychiatric team members.

The kind of psychological intervention selected for hospitalized amputees depends on the patient's medical condition, the training and available time of the potential therapist, and the motivation of the patient for such meetings. We schedule periodic visits at least twice a week after the amputation. In these sessions, the patient is encouraged to talk about how he or she feels. Some of the issues mentioned above can be discussed in depth. Some patients minimize the psychological impact through the defense of denial and may tolerate only a brief visit to "see how I'm doing." Others understand the injury has been a major life event and loss, and that at least a short-term psychotherapy will help "work through" and integrate the experience into their lives. It may be worthwhile in such situations to agree to meet on a regular basis twice a week or for a set number of sessions as described in the section on time-limited psychotherapy in Chapter 5.

For many patients, the psychological intervention is mainly supportive. This approach may allow them to express and vent feelings of loss and humiliation. It may give patients the opportunity to discuss how they are going to face people and situations in the future. The greatest benefit of the psychological intervention may be to reinforce the persons' own observations that they are able to cope well in difficult situations.

For some, the major psychological interaction may be to help them accept the idea that they could benefit from a referral for therapy sessions after discharge. Getting a patient to see the need for further intervention can be a worthwhile accomplishment and, as described earlier, there should be detailed attention to making an appropriate referral. It may take many months after amputation for a patient to acknowledge the impact of the loss, but the positive contact with a mental health team in the hospital allows the patient to take a step toward additional help.

The effect that amputations have on the surgeons and the nurses caring for the patient often necessitates interventions from the mental health team members so that these experiences do not accumulate into a load of potentially damaging baggage. Every trauma team needs a forum for the discharge of negative emotions associated with amputations. (See Chapter 11, "Care and Support of the Staff.")

Replantation

Replantation surgery—the surgical reattachment of a severed limb or body part to its original site—has become more common since Malt first reported the successful replantation of the arm of a 12-year-old boy injured in a train accident in 1964 (20). Since then, the surgery has become available at large, specialized centers around the country. The surgical procedure itself is lengthy, involving the stabilization of bones, rejoining of vessels, and repair of tendons and tiny blood vessels. The skills of at least one highly trained plastic surgeon are necessary for the success of the surgery. A tremendous investment of time, money, and resources goes into the long recovery and rehabilitation of replantation patients.

Although the larger portion of the literature on replantation is about the surgery itself, interest in the psychosocial adjustment of replantation patients is growing.

In a 2-year study of 50 replantation patients, Schweitzer et al. described the psychological processes related to replantation in five stages: preaccident period, initial response, stage of uncertainty, recognition of loss, and acceptance and reintegration (21).

PSYCHOLOGICAL PROCESSES RELATED TO REPLANTATION

Preaccident

A preaccident stressful situation is often cited in the literature as an precursor to an accident and has been discussed in this book. Use of drugs or alcohol, obviously, also increases the likelihood of accidental injury, and psychiatric conditions such as hallucinations or psychosis certainly increase chances for bodily harm. In the Schweitzer study (21), 54% of the patients reported a stressful event prior to the injury and 28% showed signs of psychopathology (including drug and alcohol addiction) prior to the accident. Recent stressful events and preaccident psychopathology strongly correlated with an adverse postoperative emotional reaction. In our own experiences, two examples of preaccident stress prior to traumatic amputation stand out.

CASE STUDY 1

A 5-year-old child wanted to ride on a lawn mower with his father. The parents argued bitterly about the appropriateness of doing this and the father won, convincing his wife that she was overprotective. When the mower hit a stump and the boy slipped from the machine, severing his foot, a spiral of guilt and blame began that affected the child throughout his replantation and long rehabilitation. This family refused suggestions for psychological counseling, and the couple eventually divorced. The child's foot had been saved.

CASE STUDY 2

A 24-year-old man was returning from a fight with his girlfriend and, in a preoccupied state, drove carelessly around a wet corner. He lost an arm in the resulting accident and had the limb successfully replanted, but continued to blame his friend totally for the injury. Issues of accepting responsibility became a major focus in his rehabilitation and failure to recover function in the limb. Only after counseling to work through his state of learned helplessness was this patient able to progress.

The antecedent of any accident is important and perhaps more so in the instance of replantation: Investment in and acceptance of the reattached limb is vital to a positive outcome. Further study in this area is needed to understand fully the linkage between preaccident stress and outcome.

Initial Response

The initial responses to burn and trauma previously discussed all apply to replantation patients. The patient frequently has a firm image of the mangled or unattached limb and a fear of being gobbled up. Flashbacks may be particularly graphic because the patient may have vividly viewed the result and retain a vivid visual image of mutilation.

Stage of Uncertainty

Fears about the physical survival of the reattached part surface soon after the surgery. Frequently, the limb must be left conspicuously visible for staff to monitor color, temperature, or bleeding, or to attach leeches that can promote blood flow from the engorged extremity. The patient becomes aware of minor nuances and perceives the crucial nature of this phase. Rigid surveillance of the limb by the patient can produce great apprehension. The staff, too, may focus so closely on that part of the patient that they overlook the whole patient as a person. Although staff members tell the patient to report any untoward changes in the limb, they often consider the patient neurotic for calling them in to assess a perceived change.

A common comment from doctors and nurses viewing a reattached limb is, "Oh, it looks great." But this bluish, swollen, functionless, insensate part may look far from "great" to the patient. Yet he or she rarely acknowledges his or her fears at this phase.

The amputation disrupts the replantation patient's sense of body integrity and, with reattachment, the sense of wholeness is often far from restored. These patients may be compared to soldiers awaiting a skirmish. They are in constant readiness and expect at any moment to have to deal with pain, mutilation, loss of limb, or death (21).

The uncertainty of this period may be a time for the patient and team to prepare for an eventual amputation. In contrast to traumatic amputations, the medically necessitated procedures often allow the patient time to absorb the reality of the coming amputation. These patients have also often experienced the reattached limb in a negative and painful way and may be relieved by at least some aspects of the eventual amputation. It may be easier to let go of a hurting, troubling limb, to make some sense of choosing this loss to avoid the ultimate infection. Amputation may be a resolution to the uncertainty of awaiting the results of a replantation.

Recognition of Loss

Regardless of replantation outcome, the patient has experienced a loss. The limb is altered in appearance and function. Reactions to loss have previously been highlighted in this book. We must note that although the family and staff may be joyous over a success, the patient may still need to process reactions to loss. Depending on the meaning given to the damaged bodily part and the patient's previous experiences with loss, this process can be difficult and overlooked.

Should the replanted limb require later amputation, it is not uncommon for the patient to feel guilt about the loss. The staff, who invested heavily in the success of the procedure, may actually feel a great disappointment that is only thinly veiled from the patient.

Acceptance and Reintegration

Because the replanted part is swollen and sutured and may at first have no sensation, it may not feel like a part of the person's body. The part could thus be rejected initially. The fantasy of a perfect limb does not fit current reality, and several reconstructive surgeries and many months of rehabilitation might be necessary before the limb is "owned." Nerves often need to be transplanted into the limb later.

Because the process of full recovery of the replanted limb is slow and staged, seeing photos of the limb at an earlier stage can help the patient and family appreciate the improved appearance. Otherwise, progress may easily be forgotten and the patient may become discouraged with the tedious process because the replanted limb never measures up to the lost image.

Families might be concerned about the patient's refusal to look at or attempt to use the reattached limb. They should be assured that patients can more comfortably look at or use the limb when they also know they do not have to at first. Patients need to have control over their reintegration and time to adjust to their condition (22).

During the most difficult parts of the hospitalization, the replantation patient may express regret about having the procedure done. But the regret is usually transient. Frequently, patients express gratitude for replantation rather than amputation. Patients with failed replants who are interviewed later are often glad "at least everything was tried" (21).

In our institution, Lee did an exploratory survey of the subjective response of individuals who underwent replantation (23). Of 68 patients who had replantations over 5 years, 40 responded to a six-page questionnaire. This questionnaire asked patients to evaluate their emotional responses during the first postoperative year and to answer questions pertaining to their perceived need for psychological supports. We note that nine of the 11 patients who felt a need for further help registered "high-intensity" postoperative emotional reaction and reported life adjustment problems. Although the majority (70%) of the patients felt that they had received adequate emotional support from the treatment team, the additional support that they thought would have been helpful was contact with another replanted patient during the rehabilitation process (23).

Good research in the area of psychological adjustment for replantation patients must continue. Assessment tools for determining who are good candidates for the surgery are lacking, and authors have not looked at the long-term outcomes for these patients. Even a more simple "Are you glad we saved the limb?" question has not been systematically asked. As in other areas of medicine, the technology is developing faster than a full assessment of the human factors.

It is clear that follow-up psychotherapy of some kind after replantation is usually helpful in facilitating acceptance and reintegration. As described above in the discussion on amputation, this therapeutic interaction may take place at many levels. The patient's contact with the transplant surgeon for surgical follow-up visits may reinforce his or her need for outpatient psychiatric follow-up.

We believe that most patients will have significant psychological sequelae to amputation and to replantation. Therefore, every psychiatric and psychosocial contact should be a building block toward helping the patient accept the idea of further psychiatric follow-up if issues of adjustment continue after hospitalization. In many ways, discharge is only the beginning of the necessary adjustments.

REPLANTATION AFTER SELF-INFLICTED AMPUTATION

The literature has some discussion of replantation in patients who have severed their own limbs. Even though the self-amputee may not be the ideal candidate for the specialized surgery, he or she should not be ruled out for reattachment. The psychiatrist will probably play an important role in the decision to reattach.

A 1980 article reviewed four case histories of self-amputation (24). This report noted that although a fair amount is written about self-mutilation such as wrist cutting, not many reports exist about those who do more serious harm to themselves—self-amputation, for example.

Stewart and Lowrey (24) summarized the types of patients who inflict self-mutilation and the apparent reasons for it:

1. The transsexual who usually confines him- or herself to genital mutilation in his or her quest to assume the physical appearance of the opposite sex;
2. The schizophrenic who may self-mutilate in response to voices ordering him to do so or out of a delusional belief that the body part is bad, possessed, or in some way hopelessly defective;
3. The patient with a personality disorder who mutilates him- or herself to relieve tension, to express anger, or to satisfy sadomasochistic urges;
4. The confused patient who is experiencing disinhibition, poor judgment, or some perceptual difficulty;

5. The depressed patient who has failed in a suicide attempt or who mutilates him- or herself as an atonement for perceived sins or anger turned inward.

Stewart and Lowrey pointed out that although self-amputation of an arm might not immediately come to the attention of the liaison psychiatrist, self-amputation of the penis certainly warrants psychiatric attention in the mind of the surgeon (24). In fact, any patient who does serious bodily harm to himself, or is suspected of that, should be evaluated by the psychiatric team.

Of the four patients reported by Stewart and Lowrey, three were considered psychiatrically well after rehabilitation. These three were employed and were also pleased with their surgical results. The fourth patient later committed suicide (24).

In another article on self-amputation, DeMuth et al. reported, in 1983, two cases of psychotically induced self-amputation of the hand (25). Although these patients benefited from psychological intervention, perhaps as important a task for the psychiatrist was to deal with the staff's reaction to the patients. The frightening, bizarre behaviors of these psychotic patients paralyzed the competence of the caregivers. The role of the mental health professional became that of reducing staff anxiety and preventing avoidance of the patient. Although the nurses were accustomed to seeing destruction, their exposure to the actual evidence of self-dismemberment was overwhelming.

Whatever the cause of amputation, it is helpful to define from a psychiatric point of view what constitutes a good replantation candidate. Perhaps the most helpful words come from Paletta, who suggests considering the total functioning of the individual as a contributing member of society and asking if that functioning is likely to be facilitated or compromised by the total experience of replantation (26).

ACKNOWLEDGMENT

The authors thank medical student Miriam Eswaskio for her help in researching information for this chapter.

References

1. Worden JW. Grief counseling and grief therapy. New York: Springer, 1982.
2. Dewis ME. Spinal cord injured adolescents and young adults: The meaning of body changes. J Adv Nurs 1989;14:389–396.
3. Selzer ML, Rogers JE, Kern S. Fatal accidents: The role of psychopathology, social stress, and acute disturbances. Am J Psychiatry 1968;124:1028–1036.
4. Selzer ML, Vinokur A. Life events, subjective stress and traffic accidents [Brief communication]. Am J Psychiatry 1974;131:903.

5. Malec J. Personality factors associated with severe traumatic disability. Rehabil Psychol 1985; 30:165–172.
6. Mayer JD, Eisenberg MG. Mental representation of the body: Stability and change in response to illness and disability. Rehabil Psychol 1988;33:155–171.
7. Ribbers G, Muider T, Rijken R. The phantom phenomena: A critical review. Int J Rehabil Res 1989;12:175–186.
8. Sherman RA, Ernst JL, Barja RH, et al. A lesson in the necessity for careful clinical research on chronic pain problems. J Rehabil Res Dev 1988;25:7–9.
9. Weinstein CL. Assertiveness, anxiety, and interpersonal discomfort among amputees: implications for assertiveness training. Arch Phys Med Rehabil 1985;66:687–689.
10. Shulka GD, Sahu SC, Tripathi RP, Gupta DK. Phantom limb: A phenomenological study. Br J Psychiatry 1982;141:54–58.
11. Postone N. Phantom limb pain. A review. Int J Psychiatry 1987;17:57–70.
12. Shulka GD, Sahu SC, Tripathi RP, Gupta DK. A psychiatric study of amputees. Br J Psychiatry 1982;141:50–53.
13. Stoudemire A. The onset and adaptation to cancer: Psychodynamics of an ill physician. Psychiatry 1983;46:377–386.
14. Lundberg SG, Guggenheim FG. Sequelae of limb amputation. Adv Psychosom Med 1986; 15:198–210.
15. Grunert BK, Smith CJ, Devine CA, et al. Early psychological aspects of severe hand injury. J Hand Surg [Br] 1988;13:177–180.
16. Grunert BK, Devine CA, Matloub HS, Sanger JR, Yousif NJ. Flashbacks after traumatic hand injuries: Prognostic indicators. Hand Surg 1988;13:1125–127.
17. Frank RG, Kashani JR, Kashani SR, et al. Psychological response to amputation as a function of age and time since amputation. Br J Psychiatry 1984;144:493–497.
18. Turgay A, Sonuvar B. Emotional aspects of arm or leg amputation in children. Can J Psychiatry 1983;28:294–297.
19. Mendelson RL, Burech JG, Polack EP, Kappel DA. The psychological impact of traumatic amputation. A team approach: Physician, therapist and psychologist. Hand Clin 1986;2:577–583.
20. Malt RA, McKhahn CF. Replantation of severed arms. JAMA 1964;189:716.
21. Schweitzer BS, Rosenbaum MB, Sharzer LA, Strauch B. Psychological reactions and processes following replantation surgery: A study of 50 patients. Plast Reconstr Surg 1985;97–103.
22. Wallace B, Chesley H. Managing the psychosocial problems associated with replantation surgery. Crit Care Nurs 1990;13:55–63.
23. Lee G. Exploratory survey results in unpublished material for a graduate program in health advocacy for Sarah Lawrence College, 1991.
24. Stewart D, Lowrey MD. Replantation surgery following self-inflicted amputation. Can J Psychiatry 1980;25:143–149.
25. DeMuth GW, Strain JJ, Lombardo-Maher A. Self-amputation and restitution. Gen Hosp Psychiatry 1983;5:25–30.
26. Paletta FX. Replantation of the amputated extremity. Ann Surg 1968;168:720.

9

Impact of AIDS

Infection with the human immune deficiency virus (HIV) results in various clinical manifestations, ranging from an asymptomatic carrier state to a fatal immune deficiency that may include encephalopathy, opportunistic infections, or tumors. The rise in the prevalence of HIV carriers and increase in the number of persons with full-blown AIDS has an increasing impact on the the physical and psychological care of burn and trauma patients.

Through June 1991, a total of 182,834 patients with AIDS was reported to the Centers for Disease Control (CDC). Of this group, 63% are known to have died, and the percentage may be higher due to underreporting. Of the reported cases, approximately 90% are male. However, women are the fastest growing group of AIDS patients, growing at a rate more than twice that of newly diagnosed cases in men. Approximately 1.5 million Americans are believed to be infected with HIV, and most of them will likely develop overt AIDS. From 1989 through 1992, it is estimated that approximately 260,000 persons will have developed AIDS.

HIV is transmitted via blood and body fluids and risk for HIV infection is related to any activity that might involve the exchange of these fluids. Table 9.1 shows various modes of infection in reported AIDS patients.

Table 9.1. Modes of HIV Exposure in Reported AIDS Patients[a]

Single Mode of Exposure	Cases Reported (%)
Male homosexual/bisexual contact	57
I.V. drug use	19
Heterosexual contact	5
Hemophilia/coagulation disorder	1
Recipient of blood transfusion, blood component, or tissue	2
Other/undetermined	4
Multiple modes of exposure	12
	100

[a] Adapted from the Centers for Disease Control HIV/AIDS Surveillance Report, July 1991.

More than 40% of AIDS patients are Black or Hispanic although these groups comprise only 22% of the U.S. population. Among I.V. drug users, about four-fifths of AIDS sufferers are from a minority group. Of the pediatric AIDS cases, over three-fourths are minority, and most are in families where one or both of the parents have used I.V. drugs (1).

Some burn and trauma units have a disproportionate number of patients who are at high risk for HIV infection. This is particularly true in urban centers where there are high numbers of I.V. drug users who may have an incidence of HIV seropositivity of up to 50%. However, the number of reported AIDS patients continues to increase in smaller urban and rural areas, and many patients who may not be known to be at high risk will have the infection nevertheless, become acutely injured, and be admitted to a burn or trauma unit. In fact, most of the 1.5–2 million HIV-positive people in the U.S. are not aware of their serostatus. Even if HIV testing were routine, results would not be immediately known. Therefore, it should be standard practice for staff to use universal precautions and be aware of the impact that HIV can have on them in the burn and trauma setting.

AIDS is a physically and psychologically devastating illness that is relevant to the psychological understanding and care of the burn and trauma patient for several important reasons:

1. HIV-related infections and their treatment can directly affect the central nervous system (CNS) and cause psychiatric symptoms as well as organic mental syndrome (OMS).
2. HIV patients may have increased rates of psychological symptoms, including anxiety or adjustment disorders or psychiatric disorders such as major depression, that may complicate the course of treatment of burn and trauma.
3. HIV infection may have complex psychological effects on the patient's family and other loved ones, which can complicate the burn or trauma patient's hospital stay.
4. The immunosuppressed state of an HIV-infected patient complicates wound healing, infection control, and other areas of physical recovery, thus prolonging an already difficult hospitalization and increasing stresses on the patient, family, and staff.
5. Medical and nursing staffs on burn and trauma units may have increased rates of exposure to patient's blood and body fluids. This often leads to fears and anxiety among staff about their exposure to a potentially fatal illness.

6. There also has been recent concern that health care workers who may be infected with the AIDS virus may be a potential threat to their patients. This point has been raised particularly in regard to the operating room and the emergency room setting.

Neuropsychiatric Syndrome Secondary to AIDS

The HIV virus is neurotropic and can be isolated in the CNS soon after the first infection with the virus.

Neuropsychiatric syndromes associated with the HIV infection include those caused by:

1. HIV itself (AIDS dementia complex);
2. Systemic diseases (toxometabolic effects of chronic diarrhea);
3. Diseases of the brain (opportunistic infections and neoplasms in the CNS);
4. Medications (agitation associated with zidovudine or AZT).

As with all OMSs (see Chapter 3), various impairments in alertness, orientation, memory, and performance of intellectual tasks are seen. Some HIV-related OMSs may be accompanied by delusions and hallucinations as well as personality and affective changes.

The mental status examination alone will not allow a ready distinction to be made between the various usual causes of OMS seen in burn and trauma patient's (as described in Chapter 3) and the HIV-related syndromes. Similarly, the psychiatric presentation alone will not allow a distinction between the OMS associated with opportunistic infections and the cancer seen in the AIDS patient. Furthermore, the degree of OMS may or may not correlate with systemic infection, metabolic derangement, or other biological insults. Also, the degree of atrophy of the brain may not correlate with the severity of the dementia (2). Patients with HIV infection are most probably more susceptible to any internal or external insult that may accelerate or exacerbate an underlying subclinical OMS.

The management of any patient with OMS is basically the same. Most important is the diagnosis of the underlying etiology. This is pursued using all available tests, including brain imaging to determine if there are reversible causes that can be treated. Guidelines for HIV testing in this regard vary from state to state and still are undergoing revision. In general, such testing is not mandatory and requires the patient's full permission as well as pre- and post-test counseling by trained and qualified counselors. With the effectiveness of AZT, and possibly of newer drugs that slow the course of the disease and its complications, it becomes imperative to diagnose HIV infection when it is first suspected in the burn and trauma setting.

The symptomatic treatment of OMS includes psychological and environmental support (frequent orientation, reduction of noxious external stimuli, pain control) and the administration of psychotropic medications. Short-acting benzodiazepines and lower potency neuroleptics are preferred. Higher potency neuroleptics (such as haloperidol) may be associated with a higher frequency of neuroleptic malignant syndrome and dystonic reactions in this population (3).

Psychosocial Problems Related to AIDS

HIV-infected patients often experience severe anxiety related to the effects of stigma and discrimination, unknown illness, unknown treatment, unlikely cure, and premature death. The patient diagnosed with HIV has experienced either a major loss of health or the threat of loss of health. The usual reaction to loss is grief or bereavement (2). Psychological adaptation may be complicated by a diminished cognitive capacity and some degree of OMS.

At the time of traumatic injury, the patient with the diagnosis of HIV or AIDS may be at the early stage of denial or may be at a point where he or she is preparing for death. Obviously, the entire psychological process becomes further complicated when this person is hospitalized with an injury. As we have previously noted, there is often a conservation withdrawal at the time of injury. In this case, thoughts and feelings about AIDS may move to the background while concern about pain, comfort, and the details of the accident become primary. Only when the patient has physically stabilized will previous psychological issues and conflicts become apparent. It may be difficult to truly distinguish preexisting anxiety and mood alterations from the anxiety and mood swing originating from issues related to the injury and the accident.

Patients who faced a diagnosis of AIDS before their injuries may have been in a crisis of alienation and expendability (2). They may have been rejected by families, friends, loved ones, employers, landlords, and health professionals prior to injury. Suicidal thoughts may have been predominant before the injury, or risk behavior that results in injury may represent suicidal tendencies. When such feelings of despair and hopelessness carry over to the postinjury hospitalization, recovery and rehabilitation may be seriously hindered.

CASE STUDY

A 26-year-old woman with three young children was seriously injured in an automobile accident. No one else was in the car. She reportedly lost control on a curve. She was not wearing her seat belt at the time of the accident. She suffered multiple fractures, several deep facial lacerations, and a collapsed lung, but was otherwise quickly stabilized after the initial trauma. She claimed no recall of events leading up to the accident or at the time of the crash. During a psychological assessment, the woman tearfully shared that her lover had died of AIDS and that she had recently been diagnosed as having HIV infection. The accident had been an attempt to end what looked like a futile existence as well as means of securing safe placement for her three young children.

This patient's rehabilitation was extremely difficult until arrangements were made for her children's foster mother to come to meet her. The two women developed a relationship and the patient regained interest in her survival when she realized that her children would be cared for and would not have to suffer neglect through her long illness, resulting in death. The patient was enrolled in an AIDS management program, and outpatient psychotherapeutic support was arranged. The patient continued to be highly involved with her children as long as she was able. As she became more frequently hospitalized, she did not have to worry about their care.

The patient facing a potentially terminal disease needs special help to recover from traumatic injury. Without a focus for recovery—a reason for living—noncompliance and sabotage of all attempts to help the patient are likely.

Staff Issues Related to AIDS

The attitude of the medical and nursing staff is an important variable in the emotional response of the HIV-positive patient who is hospitalized with a burn or trauma injury. If the patient senses continued rejection and discrimination, depressive symptoms can easily be perpetuated. On the other hand, if the staff conveys its usual positive and supportive approach, there is a chance that the patient will regain some self-esteem.

The care of the burn and trauma patient involves exposure to blood and body fluids in the emergency and operating rooms and at the bedside. Reports in the medical literature have documented that health care workers have serious concerns about their risk of occupational infection (4, 5). Recent reports of the possible transmission of HIV from dentist to patient have fueled the public's concerns about the risk of HIV infection from health care workers. These concerns lead to increased tension and anxiety, which can pervade the patient/health care worker relationship. Attempts to assess and minimize HIV exposure in the health care setting will be influenced by this potent psychological atmosphere in the following ways:

1. AIDS is a potentially fatal illness, and both patients and health care workers will be frightened by the possibility of contacting the disease if they believe that they have been exposed to the virus.
2. There is an intense stigmatization that many people have toward AIDS sufferers because of the disease's infectious nature, poor prognosis, and the negative feelings toward people in the high-risk groups. Homophobia and a desire to dissociate oneself from the victim and blame him or her for HIV infection are common.

The largest prospective study on the risk of infection with HIV following a single occupational exposure—the CDC Cooperative Needlestick Study (6)—reports the risk of seroconversion after percutaneous injury to be 0.4%, or 1 in 250 incidents. In contrast, the risk of hepatitis B virus transmission ranges from 6–30%, and health care workers at risk for hepatitis B exposure (such as burn and trauma unit staff) should be offered prophylactic vaccination (7).

Less well documented are the number and type of blood contacts occurring during various surgical procedures, including those occurring on burn and trauma services (8, 9), and the cumulative probabilities of HIV infection over health care worker careers (10).

The risk of HIV transmission from the infected health care worker to patients has recently been the focus of much media attention. Most medical organizations and the CDC have determined that this risk is miniscule. Attention to and improvement of universal precautions will decrease the risk even further. These organizations support the position that mandatory HIV testing of health care workers and mandatory practice restrictions on HIV-positive health care workers would have far-reaching negative consequences on the ability of the entire health care system to respond to the AIDS pandemic (11).

Strict adherence to universal precautions should be a priority. The staff also should be familiar with its institution's policy and procedure for reporting blood and body fluid exposure as well as with the limitations on confidentiality and compensation should the health care worker be infected with HIV while fulfilling his or her duties. Counseling about the latest information on postexposure zidovudine prophylaxis and a system for quickly providing access to this medication should be available. Health care workers should support the development of new technologies to further reduce the risk of infection and insist on access to these medical devices.

ACKNOWLEDGMENT

The authors acknowledge the assistance of Mindy Prager, M.D., in coauthoring this chapter. Dr. Prager is an attending psychiatrist on the AIDS Management Team of Westchester County Medical Center, Valhalla, NY.

References

1. Johnson J. The AIDS epidemic. A psychiatrist's guide to AIDS and HIV disease. Washington: National Institute of Mental Health, 1989:1–6.
2. Cohen MA. Biopsychosocial approach to the human immunodeficiency virus epidemic. Gen Hosp Psychiatry 1990;12:98–123.
3. Breitbart W, Marotta RF, Call P. AIDS and neuroleptic malignant syndrome. Lancet 1988;2:1488–1489.
4. Blumenfield M, Smith PG, Milazzo J, et al. Survey of attitude of nurses working with AIDS patients. Gen Hosp Psychiatry 1987;9:58–63.
5. Link RN, Feingold AR, Charap MH, et al. Concerns of medical and pediatric house officers about acquiring AIDS from their patients. Am J Public Health 1988;78:455–459.
6. Marcus R, CDC Cooperative Needlestick Surveillance Group. Surveillance of health care workers exposed to blood from patients infected with the human immunodeficiency virus. N Engl J Med 1988;319:1118–1123.
7. Grady GF, Lee VA, Prince AM, et al. Hepatitis B immunoglobulin for accidental exposures among medical personnel: final report of a multicenter controlled trial. J Infect Dis 1978;138:625–628.
8. Panlilio AL, Foy DR, Edwards JR, et al. Blood contacts during surgical procedures. JAMA 1991;265:1533–1537.
9. Melzer SM, Vermund SH, Shelov SP. Needle injuries among pediatric housestaff physicians in New York City. Pediatrics 1989;84:211–214.
10. McKinney PW, Young MJ. The cumulative probability of occupationally-acquired HIV infection: the risks of repeated exposures during a surgical career. Infect Control Hosp Epidemiol 1990;11:243–247.
11. Open meeting on the risks of transmission of bloodborne pathogens to patients during invasive procedures. Feb 21–22, 1991. Atlanta, Georgia.

10

Care and Support of the Family

It is not uncommon to hear, early in the admission of a Burn and Trauma patient, that "the patient does not have a family." Every patient admitted to the hospital does indeed have some form of supportive network. While no living blood relatives may step forward, there is almost always someone who appears at the hospital or phones and shows concern for the patient. For a homeless person, the only "family" may be a supervisor at the shelter where he or she gets a regular meal and an Emergency Medical Service worker who was first on the scene of the accident and takes an interest in the patient. For an immigrant worker, "family" may be a group of unrelated persons who are living with the patient. For an elderly widow with no living siblings and no children, family may be the young couple living next door, a distant nephew, and the friends at the senior citizens' center. Other patients have parents, brothers and sisters, children, aunts and uncles, lovers, and good friends who will come forward to play a role in the patient's final outcome after injury.

If blood bonds do not define family, what does? A useful definition might be anyone who defines him- or herself as family (1). In fact, family is that group of individuals who call each other "loved ones" of the patient and make up a network of support for the patient. The use of the term *significant other* is well accepted in hospitals to denote partners who are not married, long-term relationships, or caring others.

There are occasions during the hospitalization when legal family bonds become important. Hospital consent forms for surgical and other invasive procedures generally require the signature of the closest relative. If the patient cannot sign for him- or herself or is a minor, the parents, spouse, siblings, or, if necessary, distant relatives are asked to sign the consent. Every effort should be made to contact the closest relative, and procedures specific for each hospital must be followed in obtaining consents that meet legal requirements.

The literature on family systems often discusses family interaction patterns as being either functional or dysfunctional (1, 2). The functional family is at one end of the continuum of family styles and is marked by open patterns of communication, mutual trust, and positive support for members. The dysfunctional family is at the other end of the continuum and is characterized by closed patterns of communication, emotional cutoffs, conflictual relationships, and lack of trust between members. Although knowledge about patterns of family interaction is useful, the labels are not particularly helpful. The family is whatever it is. Most important, the family carries with it a prescribed set of experiences, coping skills, and rules that will be utilized for better and for worse during the crisis. The status quo needs to be supported in a crisis, and an acute injury is not the time to begin to change family dynamics (1). The job of the mental health team and other staff members in relation to the family is three-fold:

1. To help the family find an equilibrium in the period of adjustment to the loved one's immediate injury;
2. To assess family strengths and weaknesses and to maximize the former while minimizing the latter while mobilizing support for the patient's recovery;
3. To prepare the family for the discharge and long-term readjustment of the patient within the context of the family.

A fourth goal is desirable although not always attainable:

4. To increase the likelihood of the patient/family emerging from a disruptive and painful life experience with increased self-confidence, trust, and an expanded repertoire of coping skills for dealing with future crises.

Evaluation of the Family System

It is widely accepted that, in a family, everyone and everything has an effect on and is affected by every other person, event, and thing. Thus, in assessing the family after initial injury to one of its members, it is important to understand the multiple stressors and their effects within the given family system.

In Chapter 2, "Emergency Room Care of the Patient and Family," some of the initial staff interventions with family were discussed. Once the patient has moved to the area of the hospital where he or she will receive ongoing care, the family will meet a new cast of characters. In this context, more thorough family assessments can be done.

The following questions can help plan the care of the patient and family.

1. What was going on in the family at the time of the injury?

As previously discussed, injuries are more likely to take place when a person is under stress or influenced by drugs or alcohol. Knowing that a patient has had a recent loss, is undergoing a divorce, is out of work, or has had a recent bout of depression is vital information that the patient may not have revealed. Have there been any crises in the family in the last few months? It is not idle curiosity that sparks these questions but knowledge that an understanding of the patient and his or her family may be extremely helpful to the mental health team in its work with the patient. As the patient recovers, family perceptions and information will need to be confirmed or corrected by the patient, who may initially be a poor informant due to intubation, altered mental status, or preoccupation with pain and injuries.

It should be remembered that everything the mental health team learns from the patient or family is shared in the context of a special relationship. Much of what is known does not need to be passed on to the entire team, but may be used by the psychiatrist, psychiatric clinical nurse specialist, or social worker within the special context of a therapeutic relationship with the patient and family. Patients and families in crisis often discuss things they would never reveal under ordinary circumstances. The speed with which bonding occurs in a time of crisis is remarkable (3).

2. Who are the people important to the patient, and what other family members, whether close or distant, are likely to be affected by what has happened to the patient?

It is important to know the patient's support network because the ability to predict from where support will come helps make discharge planning a reality from the beginning of hospitalization. It can be useful for staff members to mention family members by name when talking to the patient and to relay to the patient conversations they have had with the patient's significant others. Knowing about a favorite grandmother who has been ill can make it possible to report to the patient on the condition of this important family member. "Your grandmother called, is doing fine, and sends her love" can be especially comforting words to a patient fighting for survival. Information about the status of a hospitalized or even incarcerated family member may be vital to a patient.

Staff members should be ever alert to the possibility of an overlooked "victim." The sibling who is suddenly left at home with neighbors while parents are at the hospital may need psychological support. A family member who was at the scene of the accident but not hospitalized may be suffering paralyzing flashbacks at home. Such a person (even if not a family member) may have escaped injury but may be experiencing severe symptoms of survivor guilt that could be relieved by a visit to the hospital and perhaps by a meeting with a member of the mental health team.

3. What pre-existing conflicts or tensions exist within the family that may be of concern to the patient or have an effect on his or her recovery?

It is important to know, for example, that the patient has not talked to his mother and father for years or that there are children who will find out about the accident and want to visit, but who have been estranged from the patient. What has the patient's marital relationship been like in the last year prior to injury?

A former spouse or partner may appear at the hospital and have major conflicts with the patient or the patient's current partner. Divorced parents who have never worked out a peaceful relationship will suddenly be thrown together at the bedside of a critically injured child.

If the staff knows about conflictual relationships, it can anticipate problems and intervene on behalf of the patient to make available the maximum number of supports while controlling the patient's unnecessary exposure to family conflicts. Sometimes it is necessary for a member of the staff to remind the family that conflicts need to be put "on hold" and that all possible positive energy should be channeled for the benefit of the patient. Separate visiting times can be established for "warring" family factions.

Often, as a critically injured patient starts to recover, the initial unity of the family around a common focus of concern for the injured breaks down, old conflicts come back to the fore, or new tensions arise.

4. What other crises has the family dealt with in the past and how did it handle that situation?

Since past coping is readily accepted as an indicator of present or future coping, this is an important question. Once the patient has moved from the most acute phase of injury to a phase of ongoing coping, the staff will want to remind the patient of past successes and to draw on skills and techniques that the patient/family have used successfully in the past. Negative past experiences, including "nervous breakdowns," need to be known so that patient and family can be reminded that any new experience is an opportunity to learn to cope more effectively.

While interviewing families, the alert mental health professional observes interactional patterns that may be problematic or that could hinder patient progress. Secrets, overprotection of certain family members, and dishonesty may be noted.

Family Needs

The needs of families of critically ill patients have been systematically studied and generally fall into three categories (1):

1. The need to feel hope in the early days of admission;
2. The need to have access to information
   —have questions answered honestly;
   —know the prognosis;
   —know facts concerning progress;
   —be given clear explanations in understandable terms;
   —be called at home about changes in the patient's condition;
3. The need to feel hospital personnel really care about the patient.

At times, the need to feel hope and the need to know the prognosis may seem to the staff to be in conflict. There is, however, a big difference between hearing "there is no hope for your loved one" as compared to the statement "while your loved one is critically injured and very unstable, we will continue to hope with you that there is some way she can survive." The latter conveys the notion of caring while also expressing the gravity of the situation. Families will often say, "I don't have to give up all hope, do I?" Hope for recovery is seldom abandoned before a patient actually dies. Until that time, there is no point in giving up hope even if the patient is not being aggressively treated. (See also the section below, "Loss of Will to Live.")

The need to see the patient varies among family members, and the effect of family visits on the patient and on the staff will be considered later. Especially the first time that family members go into the room to see the patient (as discussed in Chapter 2, "Emergency Room Care of the Patient and Family"), and whenever there is a significant change in patient status or appearance, family members need to be prepared by a staff member for what they will see. Fainting, especially in rooms in the burn center that are kept warmer than usual for patient needs, is not uncommon for first-time visitors.

Family Coping Techniques

Although each family is different, it is possible to classify coping techniques. These are typical family coping mechanisms seen in the early stages of the hospitalization of the burn or trauma patient (4):

1. Minimizing

These family members tend to use denial and to talk positively despite evidence of discouraging or negative progress. They sometimes seem to act entirely inappropriately and may become angry when staff members try to impress on them the seriousness of the patient's condition.

It is common for the staff to begin to avoid the minimizer and to ask the mental health team to confront with reality those using this coping mechanism. At such times, the real work of the mental health team is to help the staff to avoid alienating family members and maintain the kind of consistent support that will eventually allow the minimizer to feel strong enough to face reality.

2. Intellectualizing

These family members focus on details of the medical condition, odds for recovery, medical jargon, and elaborate rationalizations that protect them from their feelings. At times, these persons may respond well to being given "homework" assignments to keep them from feeling helpless (5). They can gather photos from home that will individualize the patient's environment or make tape recordings for the patient. They may be encouraged to keep logs of letters and cards that the patient has received or to read to the patient.

3. Self-reassurance

A spouse may say over and over again, "This is the best place for his recovery" or "I know that she is in good hands and that she will get through this." Staff members sometimes hear these words so often that they start saying the same thing to the family members. Inserting the word "perhaps" or "we hope" may begin to introduce to the family member the idea of uncertainty in terms of outcome while still providing reassurance (6). "Perhaps she will be better soon" or "We hope he can turn the corner toward recovery soon."

4. Acting Strong

Often the person who is "acting strong" is most carefully defending against a fragile interior. The person's need to know that "strong" may mean crying or releasing emotions and that "strong" does not mean eliminating all feelings but, rather, experiencing and acknowledging them. Emotions during crisis often come in waves. Letting feelings out can be the most vital part of the process of gathering strength for the next high wave. Guilt ridden families sometimes need to be reminded that there are no *wrong* feelings.

5. Remaining Near the Patient

Some family members are only able to cope when they see their loved one. These persons may have relied on the patient for stability or may gather strength from the patient by being in his or her presence. Other family members can cope adequately except when confronted with the visual reality of the injuries themselves. These differences can be accommodated. There are often supportive family members who spend little time with the patient until late in the recovery, but who come to the hospital and lend emotional support to the family members who do go into the patient's room. (See section on "Family Visits" to follow.)

SPOUSES OF INJURED PATIENTS

The psychological responses of spouses to acute burn injury have been studied by Reddish and Blumenfield (7, 8). They looked at the behavioral responses of wives of 25 consecutive burn patients and retrospectively analyzed and categorized the interactional styles in terms of the manner in which each spouse related to the clinical nurse specialist and other members of the burn team. The three main kinds of responses were described as Poor Relators, Good Relators, and Over-Relators, with the last category further subdivided into Clingers and Pseudo-Relators. The relationship of the spouse with the mental health team or burn personnel may reflect the spouse's capacity to deal with his or her own reactions to the patient's injury as well as to the subsequent problems of having a burned husband or wife.

In the above study, Poor Relators sometimes formed an initial positive relationship with the mental health team in the immediate crisis after the injury, but then cut off contact with the psychiatric clinical nurse specialist in the unit as well as other staff members as the patient began to get better. Couples with a Poor Relator spouse spent considerable time during visiting hours behind closed doors and did not socialize with other families. These spouses tended to be less receptive to referrals and sources of assistance at discharge.

While Good Relators formed a balance of interactions with the staff, Over-Relators tended to either monopolize the time of the psychiatric team or discuss irrelevant concerns in a repetitive and superficial fashion. At the time of discharge, these spouses were less able to assume responsibilities for the patient and still preoccupied with how the injury had impacted on them.

Spouses of burn and trauma patients often find themselves surrounded by their partner's parents as well as their own parents. There may be little time for the marital dyad to be alone, share some intimacy, or discuss concerns. If families cannot work out a balance on their own, the mental health professional or other staff member alert to the problem can open a discussion of the couple's need for private time. Many spouses experience relief when the patient is well enough for concerned family members to return to their preinjury lives. A spouse may also feel alone then, or struggle briefly with the removal of supports.

FAMILIES OF INJURED CHILDREN

All children are at risk for injury, and the safety of the child often depends on the supervisory capacity of the caregivers at home (8). Kitchen and bath scald injuries account for 75% of the thermal injuries to children aged 0–2 years. Within this group, 20% are injuries caused by touching a source of heat, and 5% are flame burns (9). Countless other children sustain falls, injuries of entrapment, head trauma from auto accidents, or water accidents, to name a few of the causes of injuries. This population depends on adults for safety. So the adults, and often siblings involved in a burn or trauma experience, have varying degrees of guilt associated with the injury. The psychological support needed for parents and caregivers of children can place heavy demands on the mental health team as well as the rest of the staff.

The family needs support and education to help a child recover from injury and then navigate the developmental tasks of maturation. Especially difficult may be family adjustment to deformity, acceptance of regression, and recovery from a sense of guilt associated with the injury itself. Issues of separation are often foremost in the minds of parent and child, and every effort needs to be made to diminish the negative effects of imposed separation. Most often, both the parents and child benefit from maximum involvement of the parent(s) in the care of the hospitalized child.

Parents who are distressed by their child's injury often experience a tremendous strain on their marital relationship. Couples that normally function well together find fault with each other and compete for their child's attention. It may be necessary to point out that much of their hostility is likely to be displacement of their anger about the child's predicament. Without taking sides, the mental health professional can often intervene to ease the tensions and mediate a more unified approach for the child's benefit. In multiple studies, it is the presence of a supportive network that is the most consistent predictor of positive patient outcome. Families that fail to provide cohesive support to the patient contribute to the individual's increased feelings of helplessness, hopelessness, lack of self-worth, and depression (10).

Second only to the family, the school has a great impact on the child's developmental concept of self in relation to peers and figures of authority. The entire job of the family can be made easier if the mental health team ensures that an inpatient school program is initiated for each child and that a smooth transition back to school is aided. An assembly that talks about safety, the particular experience of the injured child, and the importance of peer support for the positive recovery of any person from injury may be arranged at the child's school.

FAMILIES OF INJURED ADOLESCENTS

Accidents represent the leading cause of mortality and morbidity during adolescence (11). A teenager who sustains a major burn or trauma is immediately concerned about the interruption of school and peer relationships and is thrown into an unaccustomed role within his or her family. Given that the normal developmental tasks of adolescence are separation and individuation, identity formation, body image development, growth in the ability to maintain intimate relationships, and achievement of an increased sense of mastery, the work of adolescence can be seriously disrupted by an acute or prolonged hospitalization.

In the case of adolescents, it is often the job of the psychological staff to help the family navigate the tightrope of demanding too little or too much of their child. There is less parental permission for regression in the adolescent in most families, and parents may become alarmed at what they see. They may have been having difficulty with their child's chosen peers or life style before the injury and look unrealistically at this crisis as a last chance to effect change in ("reform") their child.

Families often benefit from the positive relationships formed between their child or young adult and members of the staff, including general and child psychiatrists. Which relationships will be utilized depends on the maturational level of the patient and on available resources in the hospital. Staff members can be role models by their ways of interacting with adolescents and can serve as a buffer between the patient and family as inevitable tensions arise.

FAMILIES OF PATIENTS WITH HEAD AND SPINAL CORD INJURY

In Chapter 3, "Organic Mental Syndrome," a section discusses special supports for the family of the head- or brain-injured patient. It is the job of the psychological team and others to help the family understand that the behavior of the patient is not completely under his or her control and that it is not his or her fault that there is little response to interventions. Additionally, family work must be done before anger and frustration set in and before a family increasingly avoids a patient and then experiences guilt (12).

In the spinal cord-injured patient, it is our experience that patients and families do not really begin to deal with the reality of the injury and permanent losses until the patient is moved on to the rehabilitation phase of recovery or is discharged. Staff often plead for psychological intervention that will "help the patient face the reality." Time is what helps patient and family face reality—a reality that cannot be grasped in the acute hospital phase. Efforts might be better spent on helping family members strengthen their own interactions, coping skills, and resources for future support.

Family Visits

Hospitals in general, and specific units within hospitals, are constantly revising visitation policies and answering complaints about whatever rules are established. Units move from restrictive policies to liberal visitation depending on the philosophy of the head nurse, the staff, the physicians, and other influences. There is a need to evaluate constantly the needs of the patient, the family, and the staff in this regard. While flexibility is to be encouraged, the need to set limits should also be recognized.

Some patients with organic mental syndrome seem to maintain orientation more easily with the presence of a significant other. At the same time, a study of the effect of family visits on the mental status of patients showed that the visits had little effect on the orientation and cognition of the patients (13).

Nurses complain that anxious family members often upset the patient. This can be observed. Perhaps the goal then should be to intervene to help families reduce their anxiety rather than to restrict visits.

Often parents do not want to leave a child's room. They may ignore their own needs for a break or the negative effect of their presence on the child. (A child may become upset when his or her mother or father cannot hold him or her because of the nature of the injuries.) Occasionally, family members need to be given permission to decrease their visits for a time to take care of their own matters, other children, health concerns, or simply to rest. They need to know that the staff will not think poorly of them for not coming to the hospital at every available visitation time. Other families need to be reminded of the psychological support that they offer the patient and need to be encouraged to visit more often.

EFFECT ON STAFF

Nurses on Burn and Trauma teams often report both positive and negative effects of family visits (14). A family can help patients develop trust in the staff by demonstrating their own sense of trust; it can give the staff positive feedback concerning appreciation of their work; and it serves as a reminder that the patient is not an isolate but part of a social system. In addition, the family is a source of valuable information about the patient.

Families often have unrealisitic expectations of what a nurse or other team member can do or can provide, and sometimes they interfere with the tasks that the treating team must complete. Families increase peer pressure and tensions of "splitting" among staff members by comparing nurses or doctors and by letting one nurse or physician know how he or she stacks up against a "superior" doctor or nurse.

Knowing the family can also interfere with the defense often used by the staff—not getting too attached to a patient who is likely to die. This can work either way: Knowing the family can help the staff in seeing the patient through the illness and with being a part of the positive outcome. Or, knowing the family can leave members of the treatment team feeling increasingly helpless in the face of approaching death. These issues are discussed further in Chapter 11, "Care and Support of the Staff."

Families of Victims of Nonaccidental Trauma

There are more than 1.6 million cases of child abuse or neglect annually, and an estimated 125,000 children are physically abused each year in the U.S. Staff members who work in the areas of burn and trauma, as well as the emergency room staff and the personnel throughout a hospital, need to be aware of how to detect child abuse as well as how to help the victim and the abuser. Abusive parents need help rather than punishment. They are most often raising a child as they see fit—as their parents raised them (15).

The following 10 items describe findings associated with child abuse:

1. Delay of more than 24 hours in seeking treatment;

2. Physical findings incongruent with the history of the event;
3. Burn or trauma injury incompatible with the child's developmental age;
4. Forced-immersion burns frequently characterized by stocking or glove-like distribution on extremities, or doughnut-shaped scars involving buttocks and perineum;
5. Patterned burns resembling an electrical appliance such as an iron, burner, grill, grate of a floor furnace or space heater, particularly involving the extremities;
6. Burn lesions resembling a cigarette or cigar marking, especially located on the soles of the feet, palms, back, or buttocks and perineum;
7. Symmetrical pattern or "mirror image" burns of the extremities;
8. Unrelated markings such as hematomas, lacerations, fingernail markings, bites, scars, bruises, and welts;
9. Unsuspected injuries, such as skull, facial, or long bone fractures found on skeletal survey, and evidence of healed old fractures not necessarily reported;
10. Behavior that demonstrates extreme fear of authority figures or caregivers, with guarding or other protective posturing sometimes along with verbal cries such as "don't hit me."

It must be remembered that adults who abuse or neglect their children represent all socioeconomic groups and that abusers are found in every race, religion, and intelligence grouping. In a broad study of abused children in one urban burn unit, the following characteristics were noted (16):

* 76.5% were infants or preschool-aged children (mean age of child abuse victim was 3.2 years).
* 71% were Black children raised by single mothers on public assistance.
* A crying and inconsolable child was the primary precipitating factor for abuse of children under 18 months of age; tension generated by toilet training and/or a soiling accident was the primary precipitating factor for abuse of preschool-aged children.
* The child was born prematurely, was hospitalized as a neonate, or experienced some other condition that interrupted parent-child bonding
* The child had congenital abnormalities or deficiencies, primarily characterized by physical handicaps or mental retardation.
* The child was born to adolescent parents.

* A poor parent-child relationship was observed in interactions. Strained interactions and role reversals were common.
* The child manifested inappropriate behavioral patterns, such as excessive crying, clinging behavior, or apathy/lethargy during dressing changes.
* The child has a poor record of immunizations and preventive and acute health care treatment.

The staff witnessing the results of even suspected child abuse must be exceptionally sensitive to other human beings without the need to retaliate. In many hospitals, it is the social worker who will perform tasks associated with suspected abuse—interview the family, interview the child, notify the child abuse registry or child protective services, and establish a plan for the safe discharge of the patient to his or her home or an alternative caring environment. The psychological team, however, may be an important therapeutic alliance with the parents and a necessary support throughout the agonizing process of investigating the injury.

With increasing publicity being given to the issues of abuse, parents and other caregivers can be surprisingly tolerant of questions that will imply suspected abuse. Some persons questioned, however, may be irate and will reject the interviewer. This is one of the advantages of having staff not associated with the actual care of the injured child doing the questioning of parents and child. The entire staff, however, and indeed every person working with a child, need to be alert to the possibility of abuse and needs to know what to watch for without being prematurely judgmental.

A multidisciplinary team approach is needed in working toward prevention of child abuse through education that increases knowledge of child development and the demands of parenting. Resources that support parents in their role are essential, and systems that foster the valuing of every individual are needed.

Loss of Will to Live

Occasionally, burn and trauma staff report that a patient has seemingly given up or lost the will to live. This volitional collapse can have grave consequences for the patient outcome and is frequently not responsive to measures of psychological intervention used for the depressed patient (16). In such a situation, the role of the family is vital.

In one study, 10% of the hospitalized patients with burns showed giving-up symptoms including apathetic demeanor, neglect of grooming, failure to cooperate with caregivers, sweeping devaluation of the environment, and nonengagement similar to that seen among prisoners of war (16). At such a crisis point for the patient, physicians may need to exert their strong potential as authority figures and to make statements such as "You seem to have given up, but you need to know that we have not. We have every intention of getting you well with or without your help, although it would be easier with your help."

A close friend, spouse, or other family member can also have a powerful influence at this time, due to bonding and the strength of conjugal commitment. It is not the time for admonitions to the patient about not fighting, but perhaps for persistent physical stroking and quiet presence with positive words of hope. Many patients who have given up on survival will later report that they drew strength from those who would not give up. Giving such strength is a vital role for family.

Preparing the Family for Discharge

As previously discussed in Chapter 4, "Psychological Reactions," discharge is inevitably a time of mixed emotions—elation about going home and fear and anxiety about the future. Patients and families need time to discuss their fears separately and together so that feelings can be validated as normal. Both patients and families need to have talked about hurdles of adjustment to reintegration at work and school and reentry to social and sexual life and to have a sense of what resources for help are available to them if needed.

References

1. Riegel B. Families of the critically ill. In: Riegel B, Ehrenreich D., eds. Psychological aspects of critical care. Rockville, MD: Aspen Publishers, 1989:31–46.
2. Satir V, Baldwin M. Satir step by step—a guide to creating change in families. Palo Alto, CA: Science and Behavior Books, 1983:197–213.
3. Berlin RM. Attachment behavior in hospitalized patients. JAMA 1986;255:3391–3393.
4. Geary M. Supporting family coping. Supervisor Nurse 1979;10.
5. Richmond T, Craig M. Family-centered care for the neurotrauma patient. Nurs Clin North Am 1986;21:641–651.
6. King S, Gregor F. Stress coping in families of the critically ill. Crit Care Nurs Q 1987;5:48–51.
7. Reddish P, Blumenfield M. A typology of spousal response to the crisis of a severe burn. J Burn Care Rehabil 1986;7:328–331.
8. Reddish P, Blumenfield M. Psychological reactions in wives of patients with severe burns. J Burn Care Rehabil 1984;5:388–390.
9. Carrigan L, Heimbach D, Marvin J. Risk management in children with burn injuries. J Burn Care Rehabil 1988;9:75–78.
10. Blakeney P, Herndon DN, Desai MH, et al. Long-term psychosocial adjustment following burn injury. J Burn Care Rehabil 1988;9:661–665.

11. Slater E, Rubenstein E. Family coping with trauma in adolescents. Psychiatr Ann 1987;12:786–790.
12. Bourdon S. Psychological impact of neurotrauma in the acute care setting. Nurs Clin North Am 1986;21:629–640.
13. Bay EJ, Kupferschmidt B, Opperwall B, et al. Effects of the family visit on the patient's mental status. Focus Critical Care 1988;15:10–16.
14. Dunkel J, Eisendrath S. Families in the intensive care unit: their effect on staff. Heart Lung 1983;12:258–261.
15. Weimer CJ, Goldfarb IW, Slater H. Multidisciplinary approach to working with burn victims of child abuse. J Burn Care Rehabil 1988;9:79–82.
16. Tempereau CE, Grossman AR, Brones MF. Volitional collapse (loss of the will to live) in patients with burn injuries. Nurs Forum 1989;10:464.

11

Care and Support of the Staff

Stress in the Burn and Trauma Setting

Acute and chronic work-related stress in the general hospital has been linked to lowered morale, impaired performance, and a high rate of absenteeism as well as to turnover or burnout of nursing personnel (1, 2). The burn and trauma setting frequently contains elements of psychological stress that may be present only in some parts of the hospital. This stress has a unique psychological impact on the health care professionals who work in the burn and trauma setting.

PAIN

The first chapter was a discussion of pain, and pain must be mentioned repeatedly as a cause of staff stress in the burn and trauma setting. Bernstein has reported how burn unit staff members are torn between their self-images as relievers of pain and the pain that they inevitably inflict during dressing changes and debridement (3). Patients often reject staff for inflicting pain (2). When patients receive relief that falls short of their hopes regarding pain control, they respond with the distractibility, irritability, and insomnia that accompany pain (4). We have reviewed Perry's theories on how the inner feelings of the staff may influence the undermedication of patients for pain (5) (see Chapter 1). Seeing patients in pain can be particularly frustrating to those staff members who are able to recognize and respond to the needs of patients for pain control. It is not unusual to see conflicts between physicians and nurses or within each group concerning proper pain control. The resiliency and stamina of the most capable staff can be taxed under these conditions, and the strain is compounded by the need to carry out procedures that are painful and that require interaction with the patient while he or she is suffering (4).

DEHUMANIZATION

Pain makes up only a small part of the sights, sounds, and smells that staff in this field must endure. There is regular exposure to affect-laden stimuli, such as mutilated bodies that include damaged genitalia, amputated limbs, and disfigured faces. The high-tech nature of modern-day intensive care is inherent to the care of the trauma and burn patient. The team approach, with specially trained staff utilizing specialized equipment, can dehumanize patient care, such that the patient is viewed as a fragmented anatomical object and there is minimal warm, emotional contact between patient and staff (6). This ultimately leads to the demoralization of the staff.

The staff members use a psychological defense, creating an emotional distance between themselves and the patient. In psychodynamic terms, this is an *isolation of affect*. It may be possible to use this defense successfully during the initial contact with the patient in the emergency room or, perhaps, in the operating room, when the focus is on the draped area or the "field of surgery." The family, however, is not hidden by the high-tech equipment and there is need for regular interaction with family members. In addition, the period of hospitalization for the burn and trauma patient is often quite lengthy and may require repeated readmissions, leading to intense inter-actions between patient and staff. These interactions cannot be easily blocked out or dismissed.

One technique that can often be used to "humanize" the patient is to have the family bring in photographs of the patient and place them directly at the bedside, so that the staff can have a better idea of the patient as a functioning, vibrant person. This often facilitates more personal, humane contact with the critically ill patient.

DEATH AND DYING

The high frequency of sudden death in a critical care setting is added stress, and constant exposure to this possibility only gives partial immunity to staff working under these conditions. The atmosphere of a modern critical care setting usually includes the expectation or at least the hope that the patient can be saved. When this cannot be done, and death occurs, a certain amount of grieving and soul searching takes place. Also, a part of this highly charged, critical care atmosphere are the inevitable mistakes that lead to guilt and anguish on the part of the staff when the patient dies (2, 7).

IDENTIFICATION WITH AND REACTIONS TO THE PATIENT

The stress of the staff may be intensified when the patient acts in a provocative and demanding manner. Some of these issues were discussed earlier, in the chapter, "Psychological Reactions." Patients who are injured and helpless show psychological regression, and the staff must be prepared for this behavior. The patient may have a preexisting history of mental illness, personality problems, substance abuse—including alcoholism—or a combination of these. Such conditions occurred in almost half of a large group of burn patients studied (8).

The stressors of the burn and trauma setting on the staff often allow staff members to have a special understanding of the psychological nature of their patient. The raw emotions brought out in a sudden painful confrontation with death and mutilation can cross boundaries and be at least partially shared by the health care worker. The staff is often able to understand the nature of the patient's conflicts and relationships with significant others. And staff often become very meaningful to the patient, even as objects on whom past and present conflicts are played out.

The occasional, complete helplessness and dependence of the patient and the nature of certain kinds of care that require regular dressing changes as well as the usual nursing duties bring a physical and psychological closeness. The frequently long hospitalizations and the readmissions to the same unit for revisions and follow-up surgery can bring about an intense relationship between patient and staff.

The psychological impact on the health care professionals working with severely injured patients is always greater if the professionals identify with the patient. Some circumstances facilitate identification—for example, if the patient and the health care worker are in the same age range or have similar backgrounds. Different patients remind a health care worker of important people in their lives—parents, siblings, grandparents, and so forth. Caregivers who are parents may particularly identify with children who could have been "their own."

Patients also experience the staff as if they were important people in their lives, especially as parents. This "transference" may facilitate a similar "countertransference" reaction by the staff. For example, a helpless patient in pain wants nurturing. The staff assumes the parenting role and makes demands on the patient to become the equivalent of a good, compliant child. If the patient does not respond, the staff person may feel rejection and anger and may act on it by developing some kind of punishment behavior toward the patient (6). For the staff, transference and countertransference can recreate emotionally laden situations that make them feel very uncomfortable, although they are unaware of the cause of the discomfort.

HOSPITAL STRUCTURE

Another source of staff stress that we must not underestimate comes from the hospital structure itself. Nurses particularly, but all staff, can get caught in the middle of clinical and patient demands on the one hand, and administrative demands over staffing and scheduling on the other. An administrative decision to float a nurse out of the unit because of a drop in census may not account for the nurse's emotional need to remain with other staff members who are grieving for the patient who has just died (and, thus, lowered the census).

Staff shortages can lead to constant overtime work demands and expectations that conflict with personal life and can cause family conflicts that spill over into the work environment.

Another source of staff stress is interpersonal conflict or "turf battles." This shows up in several forms and is especially likely when one group believes that its professional skills are not appreciated. Occasionally, in a domino effect, the housestaff feels overwhelmed and believes that it is being made to do "scut work." Senior housestaff may then pass such tasks on to junior housestaff or to medical students with the demeaning attitude originally expressed to them. Physicians may unconsciously displace their frustrations onto nursing staff. Similarly, such feelings may be conveyed within the nursing hierarchy, and then also transferred to or acted out toward physicians. The results of such interaction are intensified stress and conflict, which may lead to poor performance and ultimately unsatisfactory patient care.

Staff Esprit de Corps

In many settings, the opposite occurs. The staff recognizes that the nature and stresses of its work are unique and, therefore, a strong group spirit develops, often uniting physicians and nurses. Many staff members find this spirit an important part of a career devoted to the care of the burn and trauma patient.

Critical care nurses as well as other members of the burn and trauma team often consider themselves the "green berets" of the hospital. Like the elite combat soldiers, they believe they are the only ones who can really know the stressful, phrenetic work that goes on in this area. In fact, frequently their work areas are isolated and not often visited by other staff. (This is similar to the operating room setting.) The burn unit usually typifies this isolation. Some variation of gowns and masks may be required for anyone on the unit visiting an individual patient. Outsiders, including other medical and nursing staff, often avoid visiting the unit, perhaps because of fantasies about the unsettling sights and sounds that may be present.

Interaction Between Staff and Mental Health Professionals

The psychiatrist and other psychosocial professionals who work in this setting have a multifaceted role. They obviously have direct contact with the patient. The traditional consultation role includes giving advice to the staff about diagnosis, pain control, patient and/or family management, and referral. There may be some kind of therapeutic intervention, as previously described, and usually some kind of interaction between the mental health professional and the staff. Staff interaction may be minimal, concerning the observations and recommendations made for the patient, or more extensive and ongoing. Regular rounds and participation in weekly psychosocial conferences that are described below may be part of the role of the mental health team.

Psychological support of the staff by the mental health professionals involves two different but related components that cannot easily be separated. The staff should be assisted in its task and taught how to manage the psychological problems of the patient. This patient-oriented approach has been the main thrust of this book thus far. However, the psychiatrist and other mental health professionals who work with staff in this setting can also give staff-oriented suggestions for handling the inevitable stresses. Each interaction with the staff around the patient, or any issue about the patient, becomes an opportunity to deal with staff stresses and staff feelings.

The first task for the mental health professional is to gain the acceptance of the physicians, nurses, and other health care professionals who work in the burn and trauma setting. Usually, such a person who chooses to work in this area does achieve the acceptance of the other "comrades in arms." This person contrasts with a rotating psychiatry resident or a floating nurse or social worker who may be uncomfortable and wish to be out of the unit. The regular presence of the mental health professional in the setting itself is a big step toward achieving trust. The staff needs to know that the mental health professionals understand the stresses of their environment.

The mental health professional may actually be based in the unit, with a full-time or major commitment to that section, or may only be a consultant.

WORK ROUNDS

In the classical liaison psychiatry model, psychiatrists make work rounds with a particular medical or surgical team and establish a relationship to help facilitate the process of being a consultant to a particular service (9, 10). This technique has particular value for a psychiatrist coming into a new area such as the burn and trauma section. However, many issues must be considered before this approach can be established.

First, does the medical or surgical team want the psychiatrist? The medical/surgical physician may not want a psychiatrist looking over his or her shoulder. Sometimes, a psychiatry resident may have had more medical experience and be more knowledgeable in the medical area about drugs and dosages than a house officer running work rounds. The medical team may feel uncomfortable, and this may undermine the presence of the psychiatrist on these rounds. Similarly, any overuse of psychological language or "wild analysis" can lead to a "turnoff" of the medical/surgical staff.

The psychiatrist on rounds must learn to make useful contributions in a succinct, helpful manner. Sometimes the best remark for the psychiatrist is to suggest it may be helpful for him or her to spend some time with the patient later on in the day. If this is done properly, the psychiatrist can ultimately earn the acceptance of and develop a strong working, collegial relationship with the other physicians and the nursing staff on a particular unit.

Other mental health professionals have also traditionally participated in work rounds. Their being nonphysicians eliminates the perceived threat posed by having another physician looking over the shoulder of the person running the rounds. However, every mental health professional should be cautious about offering too much psychological interpretation at too early a point on work rounds.

Work rounds allow the mental health professional to gain a perspective about the enormous demands and pressures under which the medical and nursing staff work (1, 7). Observations made during these work rounds allow the mental health professionals to appreciate the struggles among the nurses and physicians and, indeed, among the various disciplines themselves (4). Mental health professionals who have the opportunity to join work rounds can make appropriate statements within their own areas of competence at the most appropriate time. For example, the presence of organic mental syndrome can be pointed out on the spot. A suggestion that a patient appears depressed and will be evaluated later in the day can be made. The mental health professional can devise a behavior modification plan for the nursing care of a noncompliant patient, with a plan to explore the underlying problems later. Dosage adjustment for psychotropic medications can be made and drug interactions with psychotropic drugs considered. Suggestions for dealing with complex family dynamics can be made. Disposition and discharge planning can be started at the earliest possible time, or suggestions for such planning can be made to the social worker if that person is not part of these rounds.

Often, the mental health professional on rounds can determine how well previous recommendations made during consultations have been carried out and then take steps to improve communication if there are problems.

Not all hospital units are conducive to regular work rounds. Some surgeons make rounds sporadically or have very early hours. Trauma patients may be spread out on several different units throughout the hospital and covered by more than one surgical team and even by more than one service (orthopedic, plastic, general surgery, and so forth). Often, a discrete unit, such as a burn unit, is more appropriate for rounds.

Although it is often desirable for a new consultant to spend time participating in work rounds, it may not be feasible on a continuous basis. Also, as a relationship is established with the staff, regular informal contact with the staff may become more effective than the work rounds themselves. This depends on the nature of the rounds.

One of us (M.B.) spent his first year as a psychiatric consultant at the Westchester County Medical Center Burn Unit making regular rounds several times a week. These rounds helped establish a relationship with the entire staff. In the present arrangement of the unit, one of us (M.S.) is a psychiatric clinical nurse specialist, with major clinical responsibilities based in an office on the burn unit itself, where it is convenient to be a regular participant in the work rounds.

PSYCHOSOCIAL CONFERENCE

For more than 10 years, a weekly staff conference, "Psychosocial Rounds," has been the setting for discussing the psychological and social aspects of each patient in the burn unit at the Westchester County Medical Center. The rounds are attended by the director, associate director or other surgical attending, social worker, surgical house staff, head nurse, and staff nurses who rotate in and out of the conference for discussion of their particular patients. The occupational therapist, dieticians, and physiatrists also periodically attend this conference. Each patient is presented briefly by one of the surgeons and discussed by the patient's nurse. The psychosocial professionals are then able to comment on the patient and to answer any questions. Notes are written in a special book for review by nurses on the evening and night shifts.

We believe that through this conference we have had the greatest ability to influence the staff's attitudes about patients and about its own work, as well as communicate our insight and understanding of the psychiatric and social aspects of patients. The material covered at these meetings deals with the constant problem of pain control. We are able to express our ideas about pain control described in the first chapter of this book. When appropriate, psychotropic medication can be explained as it applies to particular patients. In this setting, it is more natural to discuss openly feelings about death and dying or issues such as the heroic care of a patient with a major burn. Ethical dilemmas surface and are discussed.

In this conference, we frequently review the recognition and understanding of organic mental syndrome, an important clinical issue in our work. Depending on the case material and readiness of the staff, we introduce psychodynamic thinking and convey our understanding of the defense mechanisms used by patients. On occasion, there is insightful discussion by staff members about their reactions to the patient. The more the staff sees us in psychosocial rounds, the more comfortable they become with "shrinks."

Only because the director and associate director support these conferences and are usually present do the conferences flourish. The manner in which psychological issues are discussed at this meeting sends an overt and covert message to other staff members concerning the extent to which the psychiatric opinions and recommendations and the opinions and recommendations of other mental health professionals are valued (11). In a 10-year period, we estimate that less than 10% of these weekly conferences have been canceled.

Such a conference may not be feasible for areas of the hospital where the unit structure is not as cohesive as it is on the burn unit. However, under some circumstances, it may be useful to consider a patient-oriented case conference model that we have used in other areas of the hospital as part of our hospital-wide consultation liaison activities. This case conference involves a different "interesting patient" each week who has been seen by a member of the Consultation Liaison service. We choose a trauma patient at various times, and invite to the conference a physician, nurse, or other health professional involved in the care of this patient along with the consultation liaison mental health professionals. The patient is either taken to the conference or the conference goes to the bedside. The case is not introduced in the presence of the patient, but one of the professionals interviews the patient during the conference. Then, when the patient is not present, the entire group discusses the case. Appropriate feedback is then provided to the patient.

NURSE SUPPORT GROUP

Twice over the past 10 years, we have had an ongoing weekly support group for the nurses in our burn unit that was similar to groups we have used for ICU and oncology nurses. Our groups ran for about 6 months on a weekly basis and were well received by participants.

In the group, we encouraged open-ended discussions on any subject of interest. We, as the psychiatrist and clinical nurse specialist, co-led the group, but mainly acted as facilitators to encourage discussion. We occasionally restated unclear points and brought into focus topics that were circumvented.

When certain topics were discussed but emotions that were quite obvious were avoided, we as group leaders acknowledged our *own* feelings—anger at the provocative patient or family member or sadness over the death of a brave young patient, for example. Frustration, helplessness, and guilt were often important feelings that the group needed encouragement to discuss. The head nurse, with her consent, was not included in one group. The goal was to allow freer discussion of discontent with administrative issues. Such a session may turn into a complaint or gripe session without the channel for solutions. In such situations, we redirected the discussion. Another approach would be to assist the development of assertiveness to help nurses address problems more directly as they occur. At times, the head nurse *can* be a member of the group, especially when this nurse has come up through the ranks and is well known and accepted by the other nurses. Although we chose not to use the group to teach stress management techniques, this can be one purpose of such a group.

Physicians were not included in the support groups, but on one occasion they "invaded" the session to talk over their own grief about a particularly tragic case. Certainly, a format could include physicians together with nurses. An obvious shortcoming of this support group technique is the difficulty of accommodating nurses from various shifts. Parts of the staff who are left out or who do not have an opportunity to join the group may feel resentment. Yet some staff members may not want to join the sessions.

Some sessions were held at the end of one shift so that some of the staff from each shift could attend. It is difficult to find an hour when most of the on-duty staff members can leave their responsibilities, especially in critical care. Sometimes a period can be chosen between shifts when all the "off" people can attend and some of the "on" people can also be present. Occasionally, supervisors or physicians cover the patients during the weekly meeting. The site of the meeting could also be in the middle of the unit, but a separate room probably works best.

The support group gradually faded out after about 6 months. An improved informal relationship and informal discussions between the nurses and the psychosocial team replaced the groups.

Ongoing Informal Psychological Support of Staff

One of the key elements in both formal and informal interaction between the medical and nursing staff and the psychosocial team is the validation of the staff's experiences and feelings about the difficulties in their work areas. In a study by Koran and associates (2), a psychiatrist met every 2 weeks with the staff in a burn unit to resolve issues that affect the quality of patient care. The discussion included personal interactions and conflicts related to specific patients. At the same time, a special questionnaire, the Work Environment Scale, measured the real and ideal environments. The information from this questionnaire was then used in meetings with the head nurse and medical director. This ultimately led to increased morale on the unit as staff feelings were validated. It also sparked an interest to learn new skills to develop increased competence and techniques for dealing with stress as well as an acceptance of the inevitability of mistakes.

The mental health professionals who work in the burn and trauma setting routinely provide ongoing psychological support on an informal basis. This support includes discussions about individual patients who are being evaluated or treated, and informal discussions that arise when the staff encounters the mental health professional on the unit or converses with the mental health professional before or after the weekly psychosocial conference. Certain staff difficulties recur and surface as new patients or new staff come on board.

The tendency of staff to identify with the patient and family is one recurring issue. This natural occurrence makes staff members more vulnerable to the many emotions they feel in an abbreviated grieving when a patient dies (6). They experience anxiety and guilt when things go wrong; they will feel anger in situations that call for anger and displace their anger toward people and situations through unconscious mechanisms if it is not acceptable to express anger directly. An example might be a decision to amputate a limb after much effort had been made to save it. Caregivers may not easily express anger at the patient for "not healing" or at the surgeon for "doing this job." And so the emotions can be displaced. There might be anger at the surgeons for something completely unrelated, or perhaps a conflict may develop among peers. The staff may report increased conflicts away from the hospital, with family members and friends.

The mental health professionals who work in this area are aware of the various clinical situations that stir up these emotions. Perhaps the most important task is to help staff ventilate and validate these feelings and, occasionally, to put them in perspective. The mental health professionals can help remind the staff that it is natural to feel loss and anger and can tell them about displaced emotions. The fact that others on the staff have the same emotion and that the emotion is not an unusual reaction can reassure the staff. Even though it is expected that most staff are used to such situations and can handle them, death, dying, and mutilation always have an impact on staff. Holding in emotions and showing excessive stoicism can be counterproductive (6).

The staff is frequently impatient about the slow recovery of some patients, the demanding behavior of others, and the unnerving experience of seeing painful treatments, particularly when they are performed on children. Staff members have difficulty coping with feelings of helplessness as they witness the death of patients. The impact on staff is similar to that on people undergoing a post-traumatic stress reaction, discussed earlier in this book in the chapter, "Psychological Reactions." In fact, dreams, nightmares, and occasional flashbacks related to work activities are not unusual among staff who work with burn and trauma patients, and are especially the case among staff members who work with patients who have a major effect on the entire staff.

Sometimes, group humor and daily bantering diffuse emotions. At other times, it is helpful to offer a staff person a chance to sit down and to talk about what he or she has just gone through. If there is an ongoing formal support group, these experiences may be a topic of discussion. However, it is quite appropriate to periodically convene a group meeting for one or two sessions or, perhaps, to meet with an individual staff person for such a discussion. This is not unlike the debriefing used to help victims and even emergency workers who have witnessed and experienced an event outside of usual human experience. *The approach is to encourage people to tell what they just went through; to tell how they feel; and to tell what the experience means to them.*

REFERRAL OF STAFF FOR THERAPY

In the hospital setting, it is difficult and often inappropriate for the mental health professional to interpret acting out behavior of a particular staff member. Sometimes, in a group setting, such an interpretation may come from another staff member or the interpretation may be expressed in an ambiguous, inexact manner. However, the staff is not in psychotherapy with the psychosocial team, although it may feel that it is. At times, when the staff is venting intense emotion and going through a meaningful catharsis with the mental health professional, the situation does resemble a psychotherapeutic one. Transference and countertransference phenomena do occur.

However, before a true psychotherapeutic relationship is established, there should be strong consideration of whether the staff person should be referred to an outside psychotherapist. In fact, it is not uncommon for a staff member to request a referral for individual psychotherapy from a member of the psychosocial team. A staff person asking for such a referral for him- or herself, for a close friend, or for a family member often attests to a successful liaison relationship between the mental health professionals and the staff (10). This referral, like others, should be made with care and diligence to the best possible person or clinic setting. It is usually not advisable to enter into psychotherapy with a staff member with whom one has an everyday working relationship.

SUPPORT OF THE PSYCHOSOCIAL TEAM

At almost every professional presentation during which we describe our work in the burn and trauma setting, we have been asked, "Who gives psychological support to the psychosocial team?" Obviously, many of the psychological stressors described in this chapter can also affect the mental health professionals. Although more experienced staff members have established their ability to work in these surroundings, the first venture into a new situation may have an unexpected impact on a person, and an accumulation of stressors can lead to ultimate burnout. Anyone working closely with patients in the burn and trauma setting sees things that are out of the range of usual human experience.

One advantage of working with another mental health professional is the opportunity to informally and openly discuss reactions to and feelings about clinical material. Mental health professionals should not isolate themselves professionally by working solely within the burn and trauma setting. In our work we see patients in other areas and have been involved in teaching, research, administration, and psychotherapeutic activities. The emotional impact from direct patient contact can be mitigated by these other activities.

An overly intellectual approach can distance a person so much that he or she loses a true understanding of the patients and staff with whom he or she works. Nevertheless, there is great satisfaction in examining the psychological issues of the burn and trauma setting. These activities and this book itself have been therapeutic for us, the authors, and have helped us continue our strong involvement in the area of burn and trauma.

References

1. Fawzy IF, Wellisch DK, Pasnan RO, Leibowitz B. Preventing nursing burnout: A challenge for liaison psychiatry. Gen Hosp Psychiatry 1983;5:141–149.
2. Koran LM, Moos RH, Moos B, Zasslow M. Changing hospital work environments: An example of a burn unit. Gen Hosp Psychiatry 1983;5:7–13.
3. Bernstein NR. Emotion care of the facially burned and disfigured. Boston: Little, Brown and Co., 1976:147–183.
4. Ochitill H. Psychiatric consultation to the burn unit: The psychiatrist's perspective. Psychosomatics 1984;25:670, 689, 697–698.
5. Perry SW. Undermedication for pain on a burn unit. Gen Hosp Psychiatry 1984;6:308–316.
6. Mendelsohn EI. Liaison psychiatry and the burn center. Psychosomatics 1983;24:235–243.
7. Hay D, Oken D. The psychological stresses of intensive care unit nursing. Psychosom Med 1972;24:109–118.
8. Noyes R, Frye SJ, Slymen JS, et al. Stressful life events and burn injuries. J Trauma 1979;19:141–144.
9. Levy NB. Psychosomatic medicine and consultation-liaison psychiatry in a burn unit. Gen Hosp Psychiatry 1980;2:300–305.
10. Levy NB, Blumenfield M. Supervision in consultation-liaison psychiatry. In: Blumenfield M, ed. Applied supervision in psychotherapy. New York: Grune & Stratton, 1982:125–141.
11. Billowitz A, Friedson W, Schubert DSP. Liaison psychiatry on a burn unit. Gen Hosp Psychiatry 1980;2:300–305.

INDEX

Page numbers in italics denote illustrations; those followed by "t" denote tables.

255